In the Shadow of Fame

This book explores the author's upbringing with her famous father, Erik H. Erikson, and how her parents' attempts to heal their childhood trauma through his celebrity led to pain for them and for her.

Exploring the motivations for her parents, Sue Erikson Bloland takes a compassionate look at how the drive for external recognition and fame can distort attempts to heal childhood wounds and create new traumas for children in such family dynamics.

With fascinating insights into the Erikson family life, and wider lessons on trauma, this is essential reading for all psychoanalysts, psychotherapists, and anyone interested in learning more about Erikson and family trauma.

Sue Erikson Bloland obtained her master's in social work from New York University and her certificate in psychoanalysis from the Manhattan Institute for Psychoanalysis. She has written for *The Atlantic Monthly, Psychoanalytic Dialogues, and Psychoanalytic Perspectives,* and has lectured widely on the topic of fame. She is a practicing psychoanalyst in New York City and a faculty member at the Manhattan Institute for Psychoanalysis.

Routledge Mental Health Classic Editions

The *Routledge Mental Health Classic Edition* series celebrates Routledge's commitment to excellence within the field of mental health. These books are recognized as timeless classics covering a range of important issues and continue to be recommended as key reading for professionals and students in the area. With a new introduction that explores what has changed since the books were first published, and why these books are as relevant now as ever, the series presents key ideas to a new generation.

Imagining Animals: Art, Psychotherapy and Primitive States of Mind
By Caroline Case

Relational Patterns, Therapeutic Presence: Concepts and Practice of Integrative Psychotherapy
By Richard G. Erskine

The Patient and the Analyst: The Basis of the Psychoanalytic Process
By Joseph Sandler, Anna Ursula Dreher, Christopher Dare, Alex Holder

Discovering Your Couple Sexual Style: Sharing Desire, Pleasure and Satisfaction
By Barry W. McCarthy and Emily McCarthy

Principia Amoris: The New Science of Love
By John Mordechai Gottman

In the Shadow of Fame: A Memoir by the Daughter of Erik H. Erikson
By Sue Erikson Bloland

Praise for the previous edition

"Sue Erikson Bloland writes with keen wisdom and wonderful rich detail about her famous father, her highly accomplished mother, her family secrets, and the struggle to find her essential self in the proximity and psychic heat of their fame. I wish I had read this book as a teenager; she could have saved me a dozen years of therapy."

Rosanne Cash, *daughter of Johnny Cash*

"This is a remarkable, deeply captivating exercise in self-reflection and self-understanding. Sue Bloland excavates the complex, layered dynamics of the family that her prominent parents forged. She arrives at unprecedented depth and remarkable insights."

Lawrence J. Friedman, *author of* Identity's Architect: A Biography of Erik H. Erikson, *Visiting Professor, History of Science, Harvard University*

"Sue Erikson Bloland's memoir is, at once, a heart-rending account of family tragedy in the context of driven aspirations and profound achievement and an illumination of fame as a powerful dynamic process. She transforms pain-filled experience into personal, and now shared, truth."

M. Gerard Fromm, *Ph.D., ABPP, Evelyn Stefansson Nef Director, Erikson Institute for Education and Research, Austen Riggs Center*

"Drawing on often painful experiences as the child of celebrated parents, Sue Erikson Bloland illuminates how fame affects the dazzled public, those closest to the celebrity, and the celebrity himself."

Howard Gardner, *author of* Changing Minds, *Hobbs Professor of Education and Cognition, Harvard Graduate School of Education*

In the Shadow of Fame

A Memoir by the Daughter of Erik H. Erikson

Classic Edition

Sue Erikson Bloland

Routledge
Taylor & Francis Group
LONDON AND NEW YORK

Designed cover image: Sue Erikson Bloland

Classic Edition published 2027
by Routledge
4 Park Square, Milton Park, Abingdon, Oxon OX14 4RN

and by Routledge
605 Third Avenue, New York, NY 10158

Routledge is an imprint of the Taylor & Francis Group, an informa business

British Library Cataloguing-in-Publication Data
A catalogue record for this book is available from the British Library

ISBN: 978-1-041-08516-4 (hbk)
ISBN: 978-1-041-08416-7 (pbk)
ISBN: 978-1-003-64575-7 (ebk)

DOI: 10.4324/9781003645757

Typeset in Times New Roman
by KnowledgeWorks Global Ltd.

To Bob

Contents

Foreword to the Classic Edition

Sue Erikson Bloland is a psychoanalyst who happens to be the daughter of one of the most famous psychoanalysts of the 20th century, Erik Erikson. Her memoir dares to expose what only she could have known about her iconic father: the problem of his dissociative incoherence regarding his own attachment story, and the painful impact of that incoherence on her and her siblings. To make sense of herself to herself, she must make sense of her fame-obsessed, self-absorbed parents, which she does here with both ruthless honesty and tender compassion.

Bloland's memoir gives us an inspiring illustration of where a successful psychoanalytic process should lead: to the courage to tell the truth, in all its complexity; the successful mourning and acceptance of loss; the consolidation of faith and trust in oneself; and the deepening of one's capacity for empathy, compassion, and love. Bloland's memoir is an important gift to psychoanalysis, its practitioners and patients, by whom I hope it will be widely read.

Daniel Shaw, Author, *Traumatic Narcissism Theory: A Contemporary Introduction*

Acknowledgments

The acknowledgements which accompanied the original edition of *In the Shadow of Fame* expressed my appreciation to the people who had personally supported my efforts as a budding author at that early stage of my career—now more than 20 years ago. Those individuals had contributed to the development of the ideas presented in the book, and, in some cases, had played a key part in my training as a psychoanalyst—a training formally completed only a few years before the book was published. As I look back on that time I still feel deeply indebted to those who helped make the first edition of the book possible.

This new edition has come to fruition at a very different time in my life—through the deeply appreciated help of a different range of people, and with the important creative input of a different publisher. It is these contributors to the new edition of *Shadow of Fame* that I wish to acknowledge here:

It was Dan Shaw, LCSW, who suggested to his own editor at Routledge, Kate Hawes, that she consider publishing a new edition of *Shadow of Fame*—an idea and an initiative for which I am, of course, deeply grateful to Dan. Kate's decision to bring the book back into print was the next step in this extraordinary chain of events. And it was then Aakriti Aggarwal, Editorial Assistant and Gayathri Umashankaran, at Knowledge Works Global Limited, who played the essential role of producing the actual book! My profound gratitude goes to all of these contributors for their part in bringing about what is a dream to me: a handsome and updated Routledge edition of my memoir*!*

As for the support system needed to help me with my own contribution to this process, that was generously provided by Dr. Susan Kavaler-Adler (founder and Executive Director of the Object Relations Institute) and the writing group she has been running, with consummate skill, for many years. What has been invaluable to me is not only Susan's sophistication as a prolific writer of psychoanalytic books and articles herself, but her unwavering generosity toward others who seek to develop their own writing ability—in the form of psychoanalytic exploration or any other literary medium. Since I have been part of the group, two very compelling novels have enjoyed prolonged group attention along with psychological journal articles.

Susan has been particularly helpful in encouraging me to find my own path through the personal family drama that has been the focus of my writing for many years. She has insisted upon the value and importance of my telling my own truth at times when I have struggled with a lingering inhibition about doing so. I feel especially indebted to her for so consistently honoring my experience.

Our writing group has recently enjoyed an influx of new members, whom I look forward to working with. But I must thank one member with whom I have overlapped for a long and enjoyable time: Darlene Staffelbach, whose own writing I find very moving, and to whom I am grateful for her insightful responses to my work. And very recently, as it happens, I have been blessed with an entirely unexpected form of guidance from a newcomer to the group: Dr. Joseph Duggan, whose extraordinary range of knowledge and insight includes a unique familiarity with the publishing industry. Joe has helped me immeasurably to understand what has been needed from me now to help give this book a new beginning. I am deeply grateful for this invaluable support.

Twenty years ago, I expressed thanks to my son Per, who might have been disconcerted by the candid revelations about his own family history which appeared in that first edition of the book. Instead, he proved eager to talk about the events and issues I had written about and was nothing but encouraging. Now, I feel an equally profound gratitude for the remarkable insight and judgment he has brought to our conversations about this new edition. His engagement and wisdom has made the whole project more deeply gratifying for me!!

Introduction to the Classic Edition

Sue Erikson Bloland

When you write a memoir, as I did, when you are 65 years old, it does not occur to you that you might have an opportunity even later in your life to revisit what you have written and ask yourself, from this later vantage point, what you remember differently, understand differently, or would say differently if you were writing your story now. Having the chance to reflect in this way on a memoir I wrote two decades ago is an extraordinary experience for me, requiring that I re-read my own words and wrestle again with emotional contradictions and paradoxes that I identified then as being intrinsic to the story of my family life and as being virtually inevitable in the lives of people who have, like my parents, achieved the extraordinary.

I am very relieved to find that there isn't much I would change in what I wrote 20 years ago: about the Erikson family as I experienced it; about my parents' shared quest for fame; or about my analysis of the psychosocial nature of fame as I came to understand it back then. Luckily, writing about the role of fame in my family life—and about the emotional paradoxes which inevitably *do* accompany the achievement of celebrity—helped free me from the preoccupation with the subject that had haunted my adolescence and early adulthood. I can *remember* now how profoundly affected I once was by the excitement in the air when my father entered a room full of his admirers; or when someone I had just met learned who my father was and asked, with disconcerting reverence, whether he or she could *touch* me. But Dad's fame no longer holds that kind of magic for me, and I think writing about it helped, paradoxically, to free me from its grip.

Of course, Dad's name no longer holds the same magic for his public either now that he has been out of the public eye for many years. People who recognize his name today may still express surprise and interest in the fact that I am his daughter, but their behavior is not transformed by the discovery. It has been a long time since I have witnessed the oddly childlike behavior that his celebrity once provoked in otherwise self-possessed and mature adults; and it has been almost as long since anyone's reaction to his name has had a transformative effect on *me*! I am very proud of my connection to him now, but his fame no longer makes my heart beat faster, as it once did.

What I have found myself still wrestling with all these years later is the paradoxical contrast between my father as the brilliant psychoanalyst and writer, and the

DOI: 10.4324/9781003645757-1

more awkward and insecure man whose personal difficulties in living prevented him from being a more deeply engaged father. He was by no means uncaring, and could be shyly affectionate in his own way, but despite all his extraordinary wisdom and insight about the emotional challenges of growing up human, being a father did not come easily to him. It was sad for him and for us that he was not able to be more fully present as a member of the family. The truth is that he, himself, had not been adequately "fathered" by his disapproving stepfather or by his missing biological father (as I wrote in Chapter 3), and neither he nor my mother had chosen to engage seriously in psychoanalysis as a means of coming to terms with the residue of their own childhood trauma. [Ftnt: Of course, what was available then in the way of treatment for early trauma was not nearly as likely to have helped either one of them as the more informed trauma therapy in use today. But I still think it striking that, after leaving Vienna, neither one sought extended help from the "talking cure."]

I have always found it hard to comprehend how so many people felt deeply understood by my father after reading his books or hearing him speak—more clearly understood than they felt by their own parents or by others close to them in real life. Why, then, did I not feel that my father understood me or knew me well at all? Even though we had, for years, occupied the same house!

A remarkable MindinMind Legacy Interview with Beatrice Beebe (February 28, 2024) has helped me to understand this paradox more clearly and to forgive my father for being exactly the person he was. I have known for years about attachment theory and Beebes' remarkable videos of mothers interacting with their babies, and I have been mesmerized by images of these face-to-face interactions. But it was the deeper discussion of attachment theory that inspired me to review what I know about my father's earliest relationship with his mother to see how that might help me understand the kind of person he grew up to be.

Basic to attachment theory is the premise that the newborn infant begins immediately after birth to become acquainted with the responsiveness of his/her caregiver, and begins to learn, just as early, how to be effective in getting the response he/she needs from that person. There is, from the beginning, a mutually affecting interaction between mother and baby which is not only visible to the trained eye in the videos recorded by Beebe, but is also detectable in recorded images of the brain waves of a mother and child interacting. These earliest interactions influence the development of the baby's brain.

I have no concrete evidence to support my intuition about my father's earliest relationship with his mother, Karla (no photographs of her holding him or smiling at him as an infant), but there is enough circumstantial evidence to make this a rich topic for reflection. As I have described in Chapter 3, my father was born out of wedlock and lived alone with his mother for the first three years of his life.

What is not known is the circumstances under which Karla became pregnant, as she was never willing to reveal those to Dad. What *is* known is that, when she became aware of her pregnancy, she was asked by her family to carry her child to term in Germany, far away from their home in Denmark, to avoid the disgrace she would otherwise bring on the family. Though she was not entirely without friends in Germany, where she gave birth, Karla must certainly have felt ashamed of her predicament as well as rejected and lonely during those first years of motherhood. My father remembered that she was "sad" for reasons he could not understand, and that she spent many hours reading books—books which he later found to be written by philosophers like Kierkegaard and Emerson. He saw his mother as being "very wise," and he always associated reading with her.

I met my grandmother twice. I was not able to talk with her because I did not speak German and she did not speak English, but we did our best to be cordial with shy smiles. With me, she was very reserved. She did not hug me, and what passed for a hug between her and my father was something I had often experienced from him myself: his way of putting outstretched hands on my shoulders and leaning toward me to kiss my cheek while, at the same time, maintaining a distance between our two bodies. There may be something cultural (European?) about this kind of "hug," and seeing my father do this with his mother made me feel sure he had learned it from her.

I have tried to imagine what Dad's earliest interactions with Karla might have been like, considering that he was not a baby she had wanted to have, that there was no husband to support her, and that being with child had caused her to be exiled indefinitely from her family. It is hard to imagine her smiling lovingly or joyfully at her infant, during that time, and offering him much maternal tenderness. It is possible she found *some* solace in relating to her tiny baby, but I'm guessing that she was most interested in detecting signs that he was alert and intelligent and would be an interesting child to raise when he got older– curious and eager to learn about the world. That was how he might eventually be able to provide her with the kind of companionship she craved. And that is, indeed, what eventually developed between them.

It is the image of my father as a tiny infant—searching desperately for a way to engage his depressed mother, and learning only gradually to connect with her by being alert and curious and eager to learn—that helps me to empathize more with him for being exactly as he was as an adult. His profound dependency on Karla demanded that he develop the mental acuity required to connect with her. And he did eventually achieve an intellectual companionship with her which guaranteed her support of him when he was older and made her proud of his career. But this earliest and most critical relationship did *not* provide him with the "secure attachment" every infant desperately needs. And it is heart-breaking for me to realize what a price he paid–you might say–for his exceptional gifts.

By his own report, Dad was an unhappy and bewildered child, distant from his disapproving stepfather and tormented by the oddly inconsistent stories he was being told about the identity of his biological father (see Chapter 3). By the time he reached his mid-twenties, he was clearly emotionally unstable—lost and without any sense of direction or purpose. And that is when he was invited to come to Vienna to meet the Freuds.

What is most extraordinary to me about what happened in Vienna (see Chapter 4) is the connection Dad made with my mother, who was much like his own mother in her keen appreciation of Dad's intellect. But unlike Karla, Mother *volunteered* eagerly for the job of caring for Dad and was able to do so lovingly, providing the support needed by someone who had never learned to be truly self-reliant. Dad's intellect had matured in ways that made him very impressive to my mother and to the Freuds (and eventually to the larger world), but there was much else he needed help with throughout his adult life, despite his stature as a renowned psychoanalyst. My mother was an experienced caretaker, having cared extensively for her own mother (as I describe in Chapter 3) and though she was often frustrated, over the years, at the extent of Dad's dependency on her, it was a deal she had made enthusiastically in Vienna and never seriously regretted. She felt well-rewarded, for the most part, by the celebrity status my father was able to achieve for both of them.

This story, starting with the struggle of a tiny infant to get the care he needed from an unhappy mother, has shone a helpful light on the paradox with which I lived as my father's daughter: the striking difference between the confident, charming and deeply insightful public figure that I witnessed my father to be in his professional role, and the anxious, dependent, child-like person I experienced in private, *from whom he was dissociated* when he was fully engaged as his public self. *Yet it was the dissociated experience of his traumatic childhood and adolescence from which his deepest insights about child development and the later search for identity clearly came!* This was the essential source of his "genius" as a psychoanalyst. And coming from a dissociated part of his past, it could not be an integral part of his adult role as a father. It has taken me many years to truly understand this dichotomy and to feel compassion for what he could not be or do as a father.

And with that forgiveness has come relief from my own ultimate fear—so intense in the years before I began psychoanalysis myself, but perhaps never completely shaken—that what got in the way of a more intimate relationship between me and my greatly revered father was something quite wrong with *me*.

And having opened Pandora's box that far, I must admit to something more that I have come to understand about my part in the relationship between my father and me: If so many people felt an intimacy with him from reading his books and engaging with his ideas, why did I refuse to do either of those things? My mother begged me to read *Childhood and Society* some years after it was published, and I never was able to do it whole-heartedly. I did not want to search for connection with my father in words that were written to communicate with so many others. The idea was deeply humiliating. I can understand and sympathize with the way I felt then—but I can also see that it was a refusal to learn about my father through a medium that was, *for him*, a truly authentic form of self-expression. He had learned from his earliest days to seek attachment by giving generously of his intelligence, and that had worked so well for him for so long. I don't think he could comprehend my need—as a child—to feel known for who *I* was, and this impasse clearly caused him pain. He would have loved to discuss his ideas with me had I been willing.

My boycott seems the more poignant when viewed in historical perspective. Some years later I was to become an avid reader of psychoanalytic literature, and eventually became a psychoanalyst myself. And what I discovered almost immediately in my analytic training was that my rejection of his books had been something of a cover-up. While I had conspicuously ignored his books as an act of protest, I had been eaves dropping for years on every conversation my parents held with visitors in our family living room, and I knew a great deal about my father's way of thinking. It is sad that I could not tell him this before he succumbed to dementia, but I simply could not have had the courage to follow in those enormous footsteps any sooner than I did.

- - - -

And now, re-reading my memoir at a time when the values my parents held dearest have come under virulent attack in the country they chose as their home and dearly loved, I can't help but feel grateful that they were spared this tragedy and the grief it would have brought them. I am also overwhelmed with a new appreciation for everything they stood for: their enlightened values and beliefs, their extraordinary social vision, their essential kindness and generosity as human beings, their delightful sense of humor(!) and with how much they sought to make the world a better and more humane place. So I'm especially grateful to have had good reason to look back now at the story of the remarkable people who brought me up.

Chapter 1

Fame and the Fairy Tale

I have been preoccupied for many years with the subject of fame. My father became famous when I was thirteen, and his celebrity has since affected virtually every aspect of my life. Dad was never well known in the way that movie or television personalities become publicly recognizable. He was a psychoanalyst whose ideas and style of writing appealed to many people outside his own field—to scholars in a wide range of disciplines and to the lay public—making him one of the most widely read and influential psychoanalysts in the world.

At the peak of his renown in the United States, Dad was thought of as a cultural icon, and his face appeared from time to time in the pages of the *New York Times* or on the cover of *Newsweek* or other widely read magazines. Because of this media exposure, he would occasionally be recognized in a restaurant, for example, where people at nearby tables would whisper to each other as he was seated, or a flustered waitress, perhaps having read his best-known book, *Childhood and Society*, in her college psychology course, would ask for his autograph. Such celebrity sightings could be erroneous, however. Dad was so distinguished looking, with his blue eyes and shock of long white hair, that he elicited attention in public places from people who weren't really sure *who* he was but were sure he must be *somebody*. (Sometimes they guessed that he was Arthur Fiedler, whom he slightly resembled, for many years the popular conductor of the Boston Pops.)

It was not the breadth of my father's reputation—the sheer number of people who knew his work—that affected me the most profoundly: it was the intensity of the reaction to his writing, to him as a person, or even to the mention of his name whenever my connection with him was revealed. He was a brilliant man who also wrote and lectured about psychological issues in a way that affected people very deeply. He was perceived as a powerful father figure: compassionate, kind, and possessed of unique wisdom about some of the most difficult challenges of being human. He was revered by his readers as well as by those who interacted with him on a more direct professional or personal basis.

Dad's public aura overwhelmed and bewildered me. Was he really something of a god, imbued with the magical powers his admirers ascribed to him? Or was he the complex person whose human vulnerabilities had always been so apparent to me? My more intimate image of him was difficult to reconcile with the public persona.

DOI: 10.4324/9781003645757-2

And to the extent that he was perceived by the public as being larger than life, his idealized image posed a threat to my own sense of self-worth as a life-sized and less charismatic human being, destined to make much less of an impact on the world. Living in the shadow of his fame, I was confronted with the challenge of having to search for a meaningful nonheroic way to be, turning to sources of gratification and self-affirmation quite different from those on which he relied.

It has gradually occurred to me that the task of creating a purposeful and satisfying life in the shadow of my father's renown is not a problem unique to me or even to those who have grown up in proximity to someone famous. It is faced by nearly everyone growing up in a culture obsessed by celebrity in which so many people are affected by the godlike images of public figures that daily loom over our lives.

We have become convinced that fame is the ultimate in human achievement—that there is no more absolute measure of a person's worth than the attainment of celebrity. We imagine that the famous not only have achieved a unique social status, but actually have triumphed over the exigencies of the human condition. The gods have smiled upon them, granting them special gifts—extraordinary beauty, talent, intelligence, wisdom—which we assume have set them free from the relentless self-doubts and desperate strivings that afflict the rest of us. They have arrived at a special state of grace.

Human beings have always needed to believe in heroes who appear to have triumphed over the hardships of life. Our current fascination with the real-life heroes whose images are transmitted to us through the modern media serves much the same psychological function as the more traditional fascination with fairy-tale heroes, whose images dominated human cultural life through the simpler medium of storytelling for thousands of years. But unlike the media-generated idols of today, fairy-tale heroes were not real human beings living in the real world. They were symbolic figures—sometimes in nonhuman form—living in an enchanted land quite different in character from the world we actually inhabit. Their heroic exploits were *symbolic representations* of man's struggle to overcome the obstacles to happiness in the real world.

The scholar Max Luthi suggests that "the fairy tale is a universe in miniature," which portrays man in confrontation with the world. The fairy-tale hero confronts terrifying dangers and solves impossible problems in a journey toward the attainment of the ultimate rewards of life: "marriage with the prince or princess, … kingship or gold and jewels." Such tales of personal triumph, told by generation after generation, inspired much the same sense of awe and enchantment in the members of traditional cultures that our preoccupation with the famous brings to our lives today. They were tales about "people who were as beautiful, wise and fortunate as human beings could be" and who "moved towards and gained an absolute worth in life."

It strikes me that media-generated stories about the famous play a remarkably similar role in our lives today. We, like our ancestors, are fascinated with news about "people who are as beautiful, wise and fortunate as human beings could be," and who appear to have arrived at the pinnacle of success. In the traditional fairy tale, it is ascendancy to the throne that signifies the greatest imaginable triumph of the human soul. In the real world of today, it is fame that has become the symbol of ultimate success and self-realization. And images of the famous convey to us what the fairy tale once promised: "that we [too] can become kings and queens, or lords of our own destinies ... that we can seize possibilities and opportunities to transform ourselves and our worlds."

But the eminent psychoanalyst Bruno Bettelheim reminds us of a profound difference between fairy-tale heroes and our real-life contemporary idols. As symbolic representations of man, fairy-tale heroes are, by nature, one-dimensional figures who lack the complexity that characterizes real human beings. In fairy tales, the difference between good and bad characters is oversimplified, making it easier for the listener to identify with the good and reject the bad. Writing about fairy tales as a time-honored medium for the entertainment and instruction of children, Bettelheim points out that "presenting ... polarities of character permits the child to comprehend easily the difference between [good and bad fairy-tale characters], which he could not do as readily were the figures drawn more true to life ..."

Because of my father's celebrity, I have had an unusual opportunity to observe the way in which modern-day fairy tales are constructed around real-life people who have achieved fame. An idealized and oversimplified image is generated by the media—with the help of the celebrity and the eagerly receptive public—an image with which people can easily identify and from which they can draw vicarious strength and inspiration. But such images are not realistic representations of human beings. On the contrary, they conceal the real complexity of the people around whom they are constructed.

It is hard for us to accept that our most beloved celebrities are as complicated and difficult to really know as the rest of us, that their personalities contain as many contradictions as our own. It is difficult to believe that those who appear dazzlingly self-confident in public or in the demonstration of their extraordinary talents can also feel frightened, vulnerable, and inadequate in their personal lives; and that the most celebrated are as plagued as the rest of us by serious difficulties in living and relating, despite their charisma, their astounding abilities, and their awe-inspiring achievements. We cherish the magical excitement and the profound reassurance that our idealization of celebrities brings to our lives, and we fear that greater insight into their human vulnerabilities will deprive the magic of its power. Is there any compelling reason, then, for us to push past this fear and look more closely at the distortion inherent in our idolizations?

When we substitute the glorified images of real human beings for the symbolic heroes of old, we pay a seldom-recognized price. No one is deceived by fairy tales into believing that a small child could literally be as brave and resourceful as Jack the Giant Killer, or that a young woman could be as uniquely beautiful and pure as Snow White or as exquisitely sensitive as the princess in the story of the Princess and the Pea. However, when fairy tales are constructed around the images of contemporary celebrities, our perception of reality *is* distorted, and we embrace a deception. We allow ourselves to believe that the people behind illustrious public images are exactly like, and every bit as admirable as, their public representations would make them seem. We are convinced that we can know the famous intimately through our experience of their appearances (or performances) in public or through the splendor of their creative works. But this is, of course, an illusion. Real human beings, no matter how attractive, gifted, or celebrated, can never be as one-dimensional—or as easy to know—as the imaginary heroes of the fairy tale. The true emotional complexity of our idols is blocked from our awareness by our powerful need to believe in such purely heroic figures.

I have always been amazed at the conviction with which people have maintained their image of my father as a person. The intimate quality and tone of his writing, combined with his personal charisma, suggested to his admirers that in his most intimate relationships Dad must have been exactly as he seemed in his books and in his public persona. Yet this image of him was inevitably more one-dimensional than a real person could possibly be. It obscured the true complexity of the man.

The cost of such distortion, I believe, is that people have compared themselves to the idealized image of my father (as they have to countless other celebrities) in a way that the heroic figures in the fairy tale never invited the listener to do. It has always been clear to me that many of my father's admirers held themselves to be less successful than he was—not only as thinkers but also as *human beings*. This awareness led me to realize how often in modern life we compare ourselves to the glorified images of the famous and feel diminished *personally* by the comparison. We are deceived into believing that some members of our species have transcended all that is least admirable in human nature to represent only the best and most sublime, forgetting a fundamental truth about what it means to be human: that we are all, including our idols, a complicated mixture of the most and the least heroic qualities common to our species. It would never occur to most people that even a person of my father's great wisdom and charisma suffered as much as the rest of us from the conflicts and contradictions that plague the human psyche.

I was exposed at an early age to the kind of fairy-tale imagery that heightens the magical aura of a public figure and distracts us from the more human underside of the person we revere. Both my mother and father loved to tell stories about their early lives that depicted them as being very like figures in a fairy tale who had transcended experiences of childhood rejection to find idyllic, romantic love with each other and to ascend together to the modern-day equivalent of the throne: fame. The real story of my father's childhood lent itself readily to such tales of enchantment, since he never knew who his biological father was, and actually imagined in his youth that this mysterious person might have been a member of the Danish royal family. How often in the European fairy tale does the hero emerge from childhood obscurity to his rightful position on (or next to) the royal throne? My parents also loved to recount how they had first met at a masked ball at a palace on the outskirts of Vienna—clearly reminiscent of the setting in which Cinderella and her prince had magically found each other.

These stories and many others, oft told through the years, delighted my parents' friends and admirers and added enormous charm to their image as a couple. But they were demoralizing to me. They so heightened the magical aura of my parents' life together, and my father's rise to fame, that they made the real world, and everyone in it, seem mundane and colorless by comparison; and it was in the real world that I needed to make my own life and find my own place. Just as confusing, these romantic tales obscured the more complicated emotional reality of my parents' past and their relationship to each other. It is not that these accounts deliberately obfuscated the truth, but that they represented my parents' way of defending against the painful memories that they had carried with them into adulthood. Knowing of the pain concealed behind the fairy-tale version of their lives, I found it difficult to reconcile my intimate experience of them with the more magical account of the road they had traveled to fame.

Perhaps it is understandable, then, that I have been preoccupied with trying to clarify the distinction between fairy tale and reality where fame is concerned. My reasons are undeniably personal. I have needed to free myself from the overwhelming effect of my father's public persona. But I have also needed a means of connecting more intimately with both my parents as real human beings (even now, after their deaths) because of the way in which their own investment in fairy tales and their public image distanced them from me. I have felt compelled to try to understand my parents better through the lens of my own experience to help me reconcile the more magical public image of them with my personal reality. This search has helped me to appreciate the complexity of the people who brought me up and gave me so much, and it has deepened my love for them.

In the process of this quest, I have been inexorably drawn to a broader examination of the nature of fame and the reality behind the public images of celebrities other than my father. What I have learned about the emotional lives of other people of renown has helped me, in turn, to better understand my parents.

What follows is an account of my lifelong effort to make sense of—and come to terms with—my experience of my father's fame. It is my hope that the story of my own struggle will be a source of insight for others who must also come to terms, in their own way, with the glorified images of the famous that pervade *all* of our lives.

Chapter 2

The Orinda Years

My earliest memories of family life go back to the 1940s, when we lived on Haciendas Road in Orinda, California. The setting itself was the stuff modern fairy tales are made of: a lovely informal ranch-style house set in the rolling California hills, with shaded patio, swimming pool, trellises with hanging grape-vines, and an expansive view of the surrounding oak- and shrub-covered landscape. A golf course in the valley below the house provided a year-round splash of freshly mowed green, even in the summer months when the surrounding hills were a dry golden brown. A large oak tree at an upper corner of our eight-acre property offered generous shade for the horses that were the center of my own existence. A separate building at the end of the driveway provided a carport for the family vehicles and bedrooms for each of my two older brothers. At the back of this structure was a shelter where the horses were fed and could retreat from winter rain. My father's study was a quaint prefabricated hut that had been set among the oak trees on a hillside just below the driveway.

The nearest neighbors were a quarter of a mile away. Half a mile to the east was a large cattle ranch that would eventually be transformed into a suburban development called Sleepy Hollow. But in these presuburban days, there were still a few mountain lions in the nearby hills. At night, we heard coyotes howl. This magnificent part of California, just twenty miles east of the San Francisco Bay Area, was still that unspoiled.

It was in this idyllic setting, where it hardly ever rained in the summer, that my nearly picture-perfect family lived and inspired awe in those around them. My parents, especially, were idealized by all who were fortunate enough to be included in their social circle. My father was then working on the book that was to make him famous: *Childhood and Society*. And though he was not yet a celebrity, he was already highly respected as a psychoanalyst and had a prestigious teaching/research position at the University of California. He also had the kind of charisma that made people hungry to know him—to become privy to what he was thinking and feeling and what he was writing about. It was generally assumed among family friends that his forthcoming book would be important, that he was destined to *be* somebody.

My father was a tall, impressive-looking man, whose thick wavy hair was already mostly gray even then, in his mid-forties. His face was open and expressive,

DOI: 10.4324/9781003645757-3

his eyes a compelling blue—set off, in those years, by a California tan. He had a delightful sense of humor, a self-deprecating style, and an instinctive attunement to anyone on whom he focused his attention. He could evoke a sense of special connection and intimacy in even his briefest encounters with others. His words were thoughtful and carefully chosen, and they were granted a special authority by his German accent as well as by his reputation as the gifted young psychoanalyst who had been trained by the Freuds. Family friends sought his advice when they were concerned about their children or confronted with the inevitable traumas and tragedies of life. And his wisdom and capacity for empathy in such situations heightened their idealization of him. But for all that, he remained a rather distant figure in this social group—never fully a part of it, but admired by all of its members.

Dad's aura was felt by children as well as adults. (He was, at that time, a practicing child analyst.) But he inspired in children a combination of attraction, awe, and fear. It was clear that he was different from other adults, that some basic rules of social decorum did not apply to him because of the great importance of the work in which he was engaged. The children of the family closest to ours, the Baldwins, remember him as a godlike figure who was sometimes charming and sweet with them and sometimes unexpectedly short-tempered. This unpredictability tended to make any chance interaction with him more intimidating than pleasurable. In fact, Ann Baldwin Williams still remembers being "terrified to be alone with Erik."

Nevertheless, Dad was often asked to play Santa Claus at the annual Christmas party given by Berkeley friends. My brothers and I watched as other children sat on his knee and looked spellbound into his blue eyes. In this role, he was enchanting. How often have the three of us heard "You're *so* lucky..." from both children *and* adults who imagined that we lived with someone very much like Santa Claus—albeit more intellectual and wise.

In truth, he was an awkward father. His irritability in those years left me unsure of what to expect from him at any given moment, but he could be very warm and appreciative of the things that were important to me, and was sometimes shyly affectionate. And I had memories of earlier times, in Berkeley, when he would tell me special bedtime stories based on a native Indian legend about the princess Tamalpais. (Mount Tamalpais could be seen from my bedroom window in the Berkeley house, and the shapely contours of that mountain suggested the form of a sleeping princess.) I cherished these bedtime stories, particularly because they made *me* feel like a princess.

In Orinda, Dad's special gesture to our father-daughter relationship was to bring me little gifts when he traveled to psychoanalytic meetings in other parts of the country. In those days, the airlines gave away beautifully designed packets of information about their planes, along with lovely little mementos of the flight. Dad often flew on thc TWA Constellation, which gave its passengers an especially impressive assortment of souvenirs. These I treasured, and Dad brought them home faithfully. They impressed me more than anything else with what a truly important man my father must be.

So I still felt a special connection with Dad when we lived in Orinda, though his preoccupation with writing kept him deeply self-absorbed.

For family friends, Dad's absorption in his work only enhanced his aura. No one ever got enough of him. It was his job to make the iced tea when friends came to spend the day around the pool, and he did this with ritual care and precision, even gathering mint from the garden to give his brew a special flair. But he usually disappeared well before the party was over, drawn inexorably back to work in his hillside study. It was difficult for him to leave his writing for long. I don't think anyone considered this behavior rude on his part. Rather, they seemed honored to have had his company even for a short time.

Mother, on the other hand, was the life of the party. She was a natural beauty who eschewed makeup and dressed casually (often in the peasant blouses and skirts she had acquired while living in Vienna, where she and Dad had met). She cut her own hair and kept it short for convenience's sake. She was down-to-earth, socially self-assured, gracious and lively, and loved gatherings of family friends. Her all-day, potluck picnics were summer weekend rituals during the Orinda years (1944 to 1951).

To me, and to everyone else, Mother's gifts seemed virtually unlimited, and the Orinda place became a showcase for many of them. It was her decision to purchase what had previously been a summer weekend house and turn it into a year-round home for our family of five—virtually with her own two hands. She herself built the first addition to the house—a bedroom for me—with help from carpenters and plumbers when it was required. On her own, she terraced the hillside beyond the pool and grew vegetables for family consumption. On the hill above the house, she planted dozens of fruit trees. Although my brothers were called upon occasionally to help with heavy lifting, Mother's work was, for the most part, her private domain.

In addition to building, terracing, and planting, she ran the household single-handedly, freeing my father to concentrate on his work. She kept the pool clean with a primitive 1940s filter system that only she knew how to operate. Every spring, she held a pool-cleaning party, when the water was drained, and family and friends gathered to help scrub the walls and bottom with a Clorox solution. It was a job we children loved. We found it thrilling to stand nine feet below ground level on the bottom of the empty pool—its character so strangely transformed for that brief moment in time—and to watch, later, as clear, clean water began to fill again the cavernous space where we had just spent the afternoon. Mother supervised all of this and more.

Years ahead of her time, she embraced principles of healthy living that are only now, half a century later, receiving widespread acceptance. Trained as a dancer before she met Dad, she knew the importance of physical activity for growing kids as well as for middle-aged adults. She saw this house as an opportunity for the family to spend hours out of doors being physically active every day. In the summer months, of course, we swam. Even my father swam twice a day, sunning himself afterward by the pool. And for her women friends, mother led an exercise class that was so popular it continued in various forms for decades after she had moved away.

Our meals were always wholesome, reflecting the newly published wisdom of Adele Davis. Never did a loaf of white bread cross our doorstep; never did a dinner begin without a large fresh salad. Plentiful vegetables (some of them home-grown) were steamed or eaten raw. A basket of fresh California fruit sat on the kitchen counter, always available for snacking. We ate grapes picked from our own vines and strawberries straight from Mother's garden. Because of her innate wisdom about what was good for the human body, we lived and ate well by the most enlightened of health standards. And when a doctor's advice contradicted Mother's own intuition about what was best for us, her judgment prevailed—as when she refused to have my tonsils removed, believing I would soon outgrow the need for such surgery. She was right.

It was during the Orinda years that my mother first began to make jewelry. She had always been a very talented craftswoman, skilled at sewing, knitting, and leatherwork. Now she began to learn jewelry making from an artisan in Berkeley, and this became the focus for her artistic gifts. She was soon to be honored at crafts shows on both the West and East coasts, and her friends came to cherish her gifts of exquisitely designed earrings and necklaces, often accentuated by colorful pre-Columbian beads. This striking jewelry, showcased by her own beauty and by her graceful and proud carriage, gave my mother a look of great elegance.

In addition to all this, my father depended on my mother to discuss with him the revolutionary ideas that were soon to be presented in *Childhood and Society*. During the late 1940s, Mother awoke early every morning, before the rest of the family, to edit Dad's writing. She had grown up in English-speaking Canada, whereas his native language was German. It was her job to transform his imperfect English into the graceful prose that was to become a hallmark of his career.

Although my mother inspired admiration in all who knew her, no one stood more completely in awe of her than my father, for whom she was a figure of towering strength and an indispensable source of physical, emotional, and intellectual stability.

And still there was something more. There was the magic of my mother's charm. She emanated a warmth, a generosity of spirit, and an enthusiasm for living that drew people to her everywhere she went, and often inspired in them a deep and lifelong devotion. Her personal charisma was every bit as extraordinary, in its own way, as the brilliance that brought my father fame. The combination of their compelling personalities and remarkable abilities gave them, as a couple, a truly magical aura.

Though they were an impossible act for *me* to follow, I believed that my brothers, at least, were quite worthy of their parentage. Kai and Jon were thirteen and eleven years old, respectively, when we moved to Orinda, and I was only six. The two of them were (and still are) very different from each other in personality and style, but as they moved into their adolescent years, they both blossomed into handsome young men, each with his own special brand of magnetism. Kai was a precocious intellectual, mature for his age, and adept at pleasing adults. He was also gregarious and very popular with his peers. Jon was less gregarious, his self-confidence undermined by the trauma of a childhood mastoid operation and a stutter that followed the surgery. But whether it was despite his shyness or because of it, he had a compelling charm all his own—enhanced by a keen sense of humor—that captivated his peers and adults alike. Girls' knees tended to buckle when they encountered either one of my gorgeous brothers.

The two-year difference in Kai's and Jon's ages seemed negligible to me because of the much larger gap between their ages and mine. I was too young to be part of their social lives and felt blessed just to be in their presence whenever I should be so lucky. Of course, we shared family meals together during those years, but I never got enough of my brothers' attention to consider myself a full-fledged sibling. Mostly, I worshiped them from afar.

My memory of that time (confirmed by photographs I still have of the Orinda days) is that somehow, in the midst of that glamorous family, living in its idyllic setting, I was a very unhappy little girl. Everything about my appearance—the chubby body and face, the poor posture, the awkward manner and dress, the grim expression—reveals the truth. As awe inspiring, as delightful and kind and loving as my parents were to their many devoted friends, as joyful as the pool parties were for all who attended, there was a family tragedy just below the surface of this glamorous existence, and it was a tragedy that had affected me more directly than it had affected either of my brothers.

Earlier in 1944, only months before the move from our house in Berkeley to Orinda, Mother had given birth to a fourth child, named Neil, who was diagnosed immediately as suffering from Down syndrome. There are some parts of this story that I remember myself (as distorted as memories of such a traumatic event are likely to be), and there are parts that were told to me many years later by my mother (whose memories were also somewhat distorted by the passage of time and the residual effects of trauma).

What seems clear is that Neil's condition was serious enough to convince medical specialists that he would not live for more than a year or two. They advised that he be placed in a facility where he could get special care. While my mother was recovering from anesthetic administered because of minor additional surgery she required at the time of Neil's birth, my father was called upon to make a quick and extremely painful decision about the future care of this child. Overwhelmed with the task, he consulted two colleagues whose judgment he particularly trusted: Margaret Mead, with whom he had worked closely for a number of years, and an old friend and Jungian analyst, Joseph Wheelwright. Margaret Mead agreed strongly with the medical experts, arguing that institutional care was not only the best thing for Neil, but was also best for the whole family, which would be seriously disrupted by any effort to care for him at home. Furthermore, she warned, if Mother were allowed to see and hold Neil even once, it would be more difficult for her to relinquish his care to others, as Margaret believed she must. Joe Wheelwright concurred and the decision was made to institutionalize Neil immediately—all without my mother's knowledge or participation.

I still have to remind myself today that the steps taken to place Neil in a special-care facility could have been reversed at any time if Mother had firmly decided to care for him herself. She was not the sort of woman who had ever allowed such an important decision to be made for her. But even when she had regained her physical strength after Neil's birth, she did not take steps to bring him home. The conflict was agonizing for her. She not only had three other children to care for, but she also had a husband who was deeply dependent upon her to take care of everything both practical and personal in their family life. This was not, in itself, disagreeable to her. She was proud of her superlative abilities as a caretaker and had a profound need to be needed. But now her role in their marriage, and in my father's all-important career, was incompatible with her sense of responsibility to her disabled child. She knew Dad could not help her to provide Neil with the special care he would require, and there was good reason to believe that Dad's career would not continue to flourish if her attention was turned away to such a consuming task.

And, in truth, there was a deeper psychological (and even more painful) issue involved in Mother's inaction regarding Neil. Her self-esteem rested very heavily upon her image of herself as a strong and healthy woman who took impeccable care of her body and gave birth to (and raised) strong and healthy children. It was a crushing narcissistic blow for her to have a child with a serious disability. Had the prognosis for Neil been more optimistic, he might have presented a manageable challenge to the maternal skills in which she took such pride, but she had reason to believe that his functioning would be seriously impaired, and his life cruelly short, regardless of the quality of his care. He represented a profound threat to the image of the healthy, vital family that was an essential part of Mother's feelings of self-worth. At the same time, she felt terrible guilt and shame about her own paralysis in this matter. It always seemed to me that the shame of her own inaction fueled her undying anger at those who had ostensibly taken the decision out of her hands.

Years later, she wrote to a close friend, "I didn't have a chance to do what I would have wanted to do with Neil," and she confided to me her continuing resentment toward Dad for succumbing to the pressure of others to make a decision without her, adding that "Erik never understood how devastating that experience was for me." But I doubt that Dad ever underestimated her pain. He was not a man used to making decisions on his own, and suddenly he was called upon to make a momentous one, quickly and independently, with assurance from all sides that this would be in Mother's best interests. Ideally, he might have stood up to the pressure to act without her agreement, knowing that such decisions *cannot* be made without a mother's participation, whether she is in a physically weakened state or not. But I think it would have been deeply humiliating to him to insist, over the advice of others, that she be consulted on this issue. He felt challenged to demonstrate that he could act independently when called upon to do so. No doubt he was trying to be protective of Mother as well as of his own needs and interests and those of his other children, but by failing to consult with her, he complicated the tragedy for both of them. Such a critical life decision cannot be made by one marriage partner for the other without damaging the connection between them. Only an authentic effort to come to a mutual decision about Neil could have protected and strengthened their relationship in this difficult time.

I think Dad must have been terrified at the thought of losing the devoted care of the woman on whom he had become so profoundly dependent. And I'm sure he felt grief stricken by the loss of this child and by Mother's acute pain. He had to have been plagued by doubt as to the correctness of his own actions. When Mother expressed anger at him for sending Neil away, he was devastated and withdrew completely from communication about Neil. Each of my parents felt terribly betrayed by the other, and each felt terribly alone.

This is how I remember Neil's birth:

> I was five, and we lived on Bay View Place in Berkeley when Mother told me with great excitement that she was going to have a baby. She was *thrilled.* And in a gesture toward me that I still think of as deeply touching, she suggested that we prepare together for this new arrival. She clearly hoped that by including me in the process, she would ease my sense of loss at being replaced as the youngest member of the family. So we shopped together for baby clothes, and kept them on a shelf in my bedroom closet, where I was allowed to handle and play with them. (One childhood friend remembers how proud I was to show her these baby clothes when she came to visit.) However ambivalent I may have felt about the prospect of a younger sibling, it was thrilling to be a part of something so grown up and (quite literally) so close to Mother's heart.

And so it was that I anticipated the arrival of Neil with a special excitement. Mom and I were to share something *very* special. I imagined that I would be *needed* and would earn Mom's love and approval by helping her with the baby's care. I would learn from her how to be a mother, and we would be close.

When at last Mother went to the hospital to give birth, I stayed with family friends and waited anxiously for news of the baby. The hours of waiting turned into days, though I have no clear memory of how long it actually was before Dad arrived to give me the news. His face was anguished. The baby, he said, had died at birth. Mother was still in the hospital, and she would need time to recover physically as well as emotionally from the tragedy. I could not come home yet. And when I did, I should not ask her any questions. The topic was not to be discussed.

My next memory is of crying in my bed in the Berkeley house and calling for Mother. Dad appeared in the doorway to my room and told me sternly that she was very tired and could not come to me. I was not to disturb her again. I had lost the baby that she and I were to care for together and I had lost the opportunity to bond with her in this special way. But worst of all, my mother had withdrawn from me into her own terrible pain. I was on my own with mine.

So we were not a happy family when we packed up the Berkeley house later that same year and moved to Orinda. The setting was beautiful and the lifestyle healthy, and there were many family friends with whom to share our new surroundings. But the family had suffered a terrible blow and had no way to heal. My brothers and I had been told that Neil had died. But there was no burial, no ritual, no ceremony to mark his existence or his passing from our lives. Our parents didn't seem to grieve so much as they threw themselves into frenetic activity in an attempt to assuage their pain. They worked furiously at their respective tasks: Dad writing his book and Mom creating, single-handedly, the healthiest home environment anyone could imagine. She needed desperately to make things *grow.*

Worst of all for their relationship and for the family, they never talked about Neil—with each other or with us. Mother acknowledged this to me much later. She went to Taos, New Mexico, sometime after Neil's birth to seek help from the eminent psychoanalyst and old family friend, Frieda Fromm-Reichmann, and she was comforted by this brief visit. But other than that important retreat, she did not discuss Neil at length with anyone for many years. His name was never mentioned in our house.

I learned years later that Kai had been told the truth about Neil sometime (perhaps a year or two?) after Neil's birth, with careful instructions that he not tell Jon or me. Mom and Dad apparently felt it necessary for one of us to know of Neil's existence and of his whereabouts in case something should happen to them. This was, of course, an awkward burden for Kai to bear alone.

Dad confided to Robert Lifton years later that he had told us Neil died to protect us from a more terrible truth. I have my own view, however, of why parents choose to shield their children, inappropriately, from reality. Most often, it protects the parents themselves from having to deal directly with issues they find too painful to confront. There is no doubt in my mind that my parents were unable to confide in us about a situation that was simply overwhelming to them.

In his biography of my father, *Identity's Architect,* Lawrence Friedman suggests that my parents considered divorce during this time. On first reaction, I found this prospect virtually inconceivable, given the depth of my parents' emotional interdependence, but Mother did tell me many years later that she had suspected, during that period, that Dad was in love with a research assistant at the University of California. She had not felt free to discuss her anguish about this with anyone, she added—not even her best friend, Carol Baldwin—because of the need to "protect Erik's reputation." I have since learned that Carol knew anyway of my parents' predicament. Dad had confided in her husband, Dwight, that he was in love with another woman and was in pain about it. Dwight's advice was exactly what Dad had known it would be: that he needed to protect his relationship with Mother at all costs. (Some years later, Carol recounted this story to her daughter Linn, who just recently shared it with me. How sad that Mom was not able to seek the comfort of her dearest friend as she dealt with this tragic threat to her marriage—especially when, as it turns out, Carol knew of Mom's suffering all along.) I don't believe Dad was emotionally capable of leaving Mom at this time. But obviously, the bond between them was sorely tested.

How was I to make sense of the fact that my parents were so tortured during these years? If Neil had died, why could they not grieve and gradually recover from this tragedy, turning to us, their surviving children, for solace? Why were they still so anguished after two, three, or even five years over something that was, presumably, in the past? Why was Neil, a phantom child, still with us, draining the vitality from our private family life? I was not to learn until I was thirteen that Neil was, in fact, still alive, having outlasted all predictions of his early demise. He survived to the remarkable age of twenty-one, reminding my parents with each birthday that the experts on whom they had relied had underestimated the potential of their child. If the prediction regarding his life span was so far off the mark, might he have done better in other ways than anyone foresaw? The implications were too heartrending to contemplate. Later in her life, my mother came to view Neil's longevity as a source of personal pride and a credit to the Erikson genes, but his prolonged survival had only heightened my parents' anguish and prevented closure of this terrible wound.

It is a profound experience for me to revisit the Orinda years now, acknowledging Neil as the emotional centerpiece of our family life. My brothers and I had been instructed, in effect, to pretend that he had never existed. Yet his impact on our lives was dramatic and continues to be for all of us. I could make so little sense of my parents' emotional turmoil or the state of their relationship. I only knew that the mood in the household was grim when there were no guests to entertain. Jon remembers the tension especially at dinner, when Dad would emerge from his study tired and irritable. I remember having frequent stomachaches and asking to be excused from the dinner table to lie down.

Worst of all for me, I developed an obsessive fear that tortured me for several years: I thought I had appendicitis and was going to need an emergency appendectomy. The slightest twinge of discomfort or pain (real or imagined) in the general area of my appendix was terrifying. In retrospect, I can think of a number of ways to interpret this particular anxiety, but the most important, I suspect, is the source of the idea itself. I had learned about appendicitis from the book *Madeline,* about a little French girl who lives at a convent school in Paris, and there gets a terrible stomachache. She is rushed off to the hospital to have her appendix removed—all alone, without mother or father. Though gifts and flowers from Papa adorn her hospital room, she receives only one visit, and that is from her schoolmates. Though Madeline is brave to the point of extreme denial (proudly exhibiting her scar to her little friends), I was terrified for her. It strikes me now that I had identified with a little girl who had been sent away from home at a heartbreakingly early age to live in a boarding school. Did I actually know (on an unconscious level) that Neil had been similarly banished from home and family? And what did I imagine was the reason for his exile? Might I be the next one to go?

Kai and Jon were readier than I was to escape the household gloom by spending time away from home with their friends. Kai was involved in high school activities. Jon turned to his peers, establishing a deep and enduring bond with a group of friends who also found their family situations difficult, and who became for each other a kind of alternative family. Our friends the Baldwins do not remember seeing much of Kai and Jon around the house or at the pool parties in Orinda, which confirms my memory of that time.

I was still too young to separate in this way. I lived in a state of longing for a sense of family life and for the return of Mother's interest in me. But I realize now that my longing only reminded her of the abandoned Neil and of her own sense of failure as a mother. In a strange way, she felt she had failed *me* by not producing the normal baby we had planned for together. She did her best to attend to me, still wanting desperately to be a good mother, but her struggle with self-condemnation eroded her fondest feelings for me. She could not like me any more than she liked herself, but I assumed (as children do) that *I* was the source of her feelings of bitter disappointment.

Dad was not able to be of much help in those difficult years. He had always left child rearing to Mom, believing her to be supremely capable in all such matters and himself to be woefully inadequate. I don't believe he could acknowledge to himself that things might not be going well for any of his three children. But to the extent that he was aware, he felt quite powerless to do anything about it. He was so deeply dependent on Mother, and so frightened by the intensity of her emotional distress at that time, that my outward signs of unhappiness were intolerable to him. He was impatient and irritable with me. He urged me not to make so many demands on Mother. And he *begged* me not to misbehave in public, where my undisguised unhappiness was a source of great embarrassment to him.

I embarrassed them all. If Mother was the very model of self-sufficiency, I represented the other end of the emotional continuum. I was needy and demanding and always wanted more of her attention. An old friend remembers me as "terribly unhappy; always complaining, always upset about something." In an odd way, it seems that I took on the role of Neil. I was the child who was somehow unable to function normally in a family in which the appearance of normality was of the utmost importance. I did not conceal the anguish that pervaded our private family life. And this did not make me at all popular at the high-spirited, fun-loving pool parties, where laughter filled the air, and my parents were admired and adored.

In the midst of all this, there was one source of great solace, and it was a gift from Mother that seems to me now to have saved my life. Recognizing how lost and unhappy I felt in our new home, Mother wanted me to have something of my own. When I began to express an interest in horseback riding, she determined to make this possible, even though she knew nothing about horses (and neither did anyone else in the family). She presented me with a loving challenge, and I rose to the occasion.

My first four-legged birthday present (when I was nine) was actually a donkey named Jenny. She was every bit as willful as donkeys are said to be, and once she had been turned loose in the corral up the hill, it was very difficult to catch her. She was my problem to solve. Mother suggested that I spend time sitting near Jenny on the hillside, talking to her and perhaps reading out loud from a book I enjoyed so that she would get used to my presence and my voice. This strategy helped to diminish my fear of Jenny as well as her fear of me, and within a few months, I was able not only to catch her but also to ride her with confidence. My success at this gave me an unprecedented sense of personal competence.

My relationship with Jenny suffered a setback when I was riding past a nearby house one afternoon, and she was startled by the neighbor's dog. He dashed out of a driveway barking loudly and nipping at Jenny's heels. The next thing I remember is hitting the road and watching Jenny disappear into the distance. My arm hurt badly, but my greatest worry was that Jenny would get away. I followed her and eventually caught her, to my great relief. After I had led her home to the corral, I went to show Mom my swollen wrist. I was in a cast for the next six weeks.

My obvious sense of responsibility for Jenny helped earn an upgrade to my first horse, named Spot, which I subsequently rode all over the Orinda hills. Mother won my undying gratitude when she insisted, over Dad's fears, that one broken wrist was not enough to put an end to my riding career. She understood how much I needed this source of autonomy and self-confidence. And she trusted my judgment and ability enough to put me in full charge of these big strong animals (even after the mishap with Jenny). She admired my pluck and determination where riding was concerned, and that, in itself, was a great boost to my morale.

Many years later, as Mother reflected back on this time, she wrote a few lines about Jenny:

> So one day [Sue] prevailed. We went and procured for her Jenny—her donkey—her very own ornery, strong-minded donkey that no one else dared ride. She made it obey but also fed, cared for and lived for it. When, it hee-hawed and scared the neighbors in our quiet valley, we pretended the voice was charming.
>
> When she really had it under control—no one else had—she rode off over the hill to the watershed lands above us and was queen of all she surveyed. My hair grew definitely gray...... Dear Jenny wherever you are braying, Bless you!

Her appreciation of what this meant to me still touches me deeply.

So eventually I, too, had a way of escaping the household for hours each day. And at that time, Orinda offered wonderful open spaces to explore. I often rode alone, but felt bonded with Jenny and the horses that followed her (Blaze came after Spot) in a way that gave me great comfort. I read avidly about the Old West and identified with the image of the cowboy riding solo on the open range. I loved being in control of a big strong animal and going wherever I wanted to go. Riding was my solace, my pleasure, and my greatest source of self-esteem. Even today I feel proud of the cowgirl I became—of my taming of the willful Jenny, of my riding ability, of my competent care for these animals, and, perhaps most of all, of the sense of independence from Mother that riding began to make possible for me.

Mother took great pleasure in my moments of triumph as a cowgirl. And she did many wonderful things for me during those years. She rented a horse trailer, once, when I wanted desperately to ride in a rodeo thirty or forty miles away. My job was to get the horse in and out of this strange vehicle, which, as I recall, was not easy. Mother's job was to drive the car up and down mountain roads, pulling a very unfamiliar load. We both took pride in our success that day.

And there were Christmas gifts so perfectly attuned to my tastes and desires that it was clear she knew me better than anyone else in the world. One was a beautifully carved Indian pony with its own exquisite little leather saddle and bridal, and a saddle blanket of Indian design. It was a cherished possession throughout my childhood, and I still have it to this day.

But despite such expressions of love, Mother could not enjoy my company the way she enjoyed the company of other people's children, including the daughters of the family that was closest to ours. She exuded warmth and affection with them, and they loved her in return, making her feel like the quintessentially good mother she so wished she could be. They, too, suffered a family loss during those years (their father died of cancer), but they did not *look* depressed the way I did and, most important, Mother felt no responsibility for their pain. And so it was possible for her to laugh playfully with them in a way that she could not laugh with me, and I was terribly envious of that. One of the neighborhood children from Orinda has recently reminded me of how much my parents did for her when her own family was in great distress. Mother was exceptionally attuned to unhappiness in other people's children and reached out to them in ways they never forgot. There was only one interpretation I could make at the time: this beautiful, talented, and beloved woman would be so much happier if one of these other delightful little girls had been her daughter.

I have heard enough family stories in my work as a psychotherapist to know that there is nothing terribly out of the ordinary in the picture I have just painted of my family life in the 1940s. Families suffer all kinds of tragedies (many far worse than ours) and are, quite typically, afraid to talk about them or grieve them together. The result is the isolation of family members from one another and the tendency for children to construct fantasies to help them make sense out of unexplained events and circumstances. Sometimes such fantasies are more devastating in their implications than the reality they are meant to clarify. For example, children typically assume that they are, somehow, the cause of the bad things that have happened or bad feelings that persist in their family life, and such assumptions go right with them (consciously or unconsciously) into adulthood.

It is also typical for families to maintain a facade, an external image, which is different in important respects from the reality of their internal life and which conceals family distress. Many clients have described to me a bewildering discrepancy between the public behavior or image of their parents and the very different behavior that manifested itself in their intimate family relationships. Indeed, many members of families in pain exhibit exceptionally bright smiles, pleasing personalities, and impressive facades to the outside world to help defend against the feelings of shame and unhappiness that lurk below the surface of family life.

I know all this now, but I certainly did not know it then. In addition to the mystery of Neil and of my parents' inexplicable suffering, as the years went by, I was also deeply bewildered by the difference between my parents as I experienced them in the context of the family and my parents as they were with friends and admirers. I had been presented with two seemingly inconsistent images of my mother and father during those years. I was aware that they were deeply unhappy, that they were wrestling with inner demons, and that there was a desperation in the way they both threw themselves into their work. In private, I experienced them as emotionally fragile and vulnerable, and I was frightened for them, felt sad for them, wished I could make them feel better.

Then when guests arrived, my parents were magically transformed. I don't mean to suggest that they put on an empty show. They *felt* different in social settings. They felt better about themselves, more vital and warm and alive in the company of other people than they felt during family dinners. It was already clear to me in those days that their interactions with admiring friends revitalized them, affirmed them, gratified them in a way that family life could not. And based on the warmth, self-confidence, and generosity they exuded in social situations, an image was created of two exceptionally gifted people who shared a special expertise in the art of living and loving. Their public image reflected everything they most *wanted* to be, while in their private lives, they were tormented by unexplored, never-clarified feelings about their relationship to Neil, to each other, and to their other three children.

As my father became famous, my parents' relationship with each other was gradually (though never completely) healed by their mutual investment in Dad's career and the gratification they both experienced as a result of his success. Because of their obvious affection for each other, the magic of their public personalities, and especially because of the very intimate content and personal style of my father's writing, it was always assumed that they, more than most mortals, were capable of dealing directly and honestly with the most difficult emotional challenges that life and human relationships present. And this image was greatly enhanced by their mutual ability to help others through emotional crises, and by the intimacy that their friends and admirers experienced in their interactions with them. Yet the most troubling issues in their relationship with each other, or in their relationships with their own children, could never be openly discussed. We were not a family that ever talked about the things that hurt or angered us the most, which left many sources of hurt and anger unexplored and unresolved. It also left me with a pervasive fear of opening my parents' wounds and seeing the anguish on their faces that any reference to a painful issue might suddenly evoke. I dreaded the abrupt sense of disconnection from them that inevitably followed. For as long as my parents lived, I went to great lengths to avoid such interpersonal catastrophes in my interactions with them.

Chapter 3

My Parents' Childhoods

It is impossible to understand the paradoxes of our family life during the Orinda years without knowing something about my mother's and father's own childhoods and the way their early experiences related to their difficult struggle to be good parents themselves. I was very little when I first began to hear stories about my parents' early family lives, and it seems as though I always knew that they had both felt rejected as children. Although they grew up in different countries and cultures (Mother in Canada and the United States, Dad in Germany), and their families of origin were quite different in character, they shared a sense of having been misfits throughout their early years—of having felt alienated from their families and from the immediate environment in which they each lived. Mother took pride in thinking of herself, and of Dad, as having been very much like the ugly duckling of the Hans Christian Andersen fairy tale: perceived early on as being strange and different—their uniqueness unappreciated, if not actively disdained, by those around them—but discovering as young adults that the very differentness for which they had felt rejected was the stuff that swans (or human beings destined for greatness) are made of.

Their first meeting—at a masked ball in Vienna—was itself like a fairy tale. Almost instantly, they recognized in each other the extraordinary qualities that had been deprecated in their childhood pasts, but that offered them both the possibility of a triumphant future. In the fairy-tale version of such a magical coming together, the couple always lives happily ever after. In my parents' case, their future included the traumas and stresses that afflict most human lives and relationships. But what *was* magical about their union was the joining of their respective gifts, and the impact they were able to have together on the world at large. Neither of them could have attained the same level of success without the other. And most importantly, from a historical perspective, my father could never have achieved what he did without my mother. "He would have been nothing without Joan," his half-sisters have both agreed.

...

Mother was born in 1903 in a small town in Ontario, Canada. She was christened Sarah Lucretia Mowat Serson and was called Sally as a child. Later, she was to

DOI: 10.4324/9781003645757-4

change her name to Joan. Though I don't know what drew her to that name, I was aware even as a child that she hated being called either Sarah or Sally.

A chronology of Mother's childhood is difficult to reconstruct because she was moved from one place to another in rapid succession. But the emotional tenor of those early years is etched deeply in my own memory because of the many stories she told me when I was small, and because of a series of childhood reminiscences she wrote when she was in her eighties. Her descriptions of her early family life have always touched me deeply and have helped me—more than anything else—to understand the sometimes baffling person she was to me.

The town in which Mother was born was Gananoque, on the St. Lawrence River, where her father, John Serson, was rector of the local Episcopal church. My mother's remembrance of her father is particularly poignant:

> I don't think I can get God and my father apart. They were both so far away and I respected them because everyone else around respected them both so much—about equally it seemed. God spoke to other people directly—the bible had lots of stories about this—but not to me. Father never did either, except once when I was about seven or eight. I had been really bad, hopelessly bad, and mother thought up this truly awful way to set me straight for good. She sent me into his study to confess. He took me on his lap—only time ever—and explained that what I had done was wicked. He meant so well—and I could feel that, but the warmth that could have made me feel less wicked wasn't there. I think he was almost embarrassed—I was. Poor us!!! A year later he died. I gulped at his funeral—everyone was very touched. I felt I'd lost what I never really ever had.

And things were hardly better between my mother and *her* mother, Mary MacDonald Serson. Mary was an emotionally detached and straitlaced woman, a devout Episcopalian from a wealthy family in New York City. She had come to the town of Gananoque to marry my grandfather, John; but the marriage was never a happy one, and she found herself hopelessly out of place in the provincial Canadian setting. Her profound unhappiness and sense of deprivation (never to be relieved, as it turned out) were to cast a long shadow over the lives of her children. In her written reminiscences, Mother often refers to Mary, quite strikingly, as "my parent"—reflecting the chilly distance she experienced in this all-important relationship. She describes Mary as a tough disciplinarian who "ruled all the details of our house and our lives, and I mean *ruled.*" Mary's primary interest as a mother was the molding of clean, neat, and obedient children. Mother was the youngest of the three children who were expected to uphold this unnatural standard, and she was the least successful at it. Her older brother, Don, could be mischievous in play with his sisters, but was good at maintaining decorum in the presence of his parents. The middle child, Molly, two years older than my mother, was a veritable angel—always the good one, preferred and generously rewarded by both parents. "Molly got first choice on everything because she was two years older—and of course she was good, so good, and I was always in trouble." Mother was not only in frequent trouble, but she was viewed as a hopelessly wicked child. Addressing her mother in a memoir (many years after Mary's death), she wrote, "You made me feel 'bad,' not just naughty but really somehow bad and selfish and secretive and of course stubborn ... I so admired you and longed for more intimacy. You were very fine and far away." And in one three-sentence sketch entitled "Hateful Memory," Mother wrote, "I took her my first poem. She read it and thanked me—said it was nice. Later I overheard her say to Grandfather, 'She probably copied it from somewhere.'"

Mother felt so hopelessly rejected by Mary that she worked hard to hide her longing for Mary's love and admiration. She deeply envied Molly's position in the family as their mother's pet. But it was quite impossible for her to compete with Molly's unerring "goodness." Mother describes herself as a "secretive, envious, and miserable" child who yearned for praise and hid her misery behind bravura so no one would see how devastated she felt. She took special pride in being courageous and self-reliant—a desperate effort to convince herself (and others) through her bravado that she was afraid of nothing and did not *need* parental approval or care. She frequently engaged in secretive (and seemingly rather dangerous) adventures all by herself: "I would sail off in my small dinghy quite alone and try the rough parts of the lake out toward the Granite Tomb, then head into a small half-wooded island and spend hours there exploring, swimming off the rocks and drying naked in the sun .... "

Thinking back to the years of her childhood, Mother exclaims about herself, "What a loner!" but continues, wistfully, "I think often a lonely loner." She confessed that she could not remember having a single friend until she was eleven or twelve years old. And even then, when she and a neighbor began to ride their bicycles together, they talked about nothing personal. It was exciting for Mother to have a companion willing to take "risky" rides with her into "forbidden territory," but she could remember no moments of intimacy in this relationship, and continued to feel emotionally isolated.

I am especially touched by Mother's account of slipping and banging her head on some stone steps when she was five or six and being taken to the doctor to have the wound stitched up.

> He was a nice doctor ... I did just what he said and was so quiet. He kept exclaiming about how brave I was. I was inflated with bravery.
>
> When I left, he patted me and gave me a lovely doll in a peasant costume, with lots more words about how remarkably brave I had been.

Looking on as her daughter received such praise, Mary just seemed perplexed, as though she could not imagine what this doctor found so admirable about her rebellious little girl. How sad that Mother's only comfort came from the doctor. And how sad that Mother's desperate need for praise made this experience one of her *happy* memories. This vignette illustrates the way she had dealt with the total lack of warmth and support from Mary by becoming remarkably courageous for such a little girl.

But there was one person from whom Mother *did* get love and approval in her early childhood years. Her maternal grandmother, whom she called Nama, felt a deep connection with her and admired her intelligence as well as her bold and mischievous spirit. She made Mother feel like a very special child, whose remarkable qualities would one day be widely recognized and appreciated. Nama was a source of vital emotional nourishment for Mother in an otherwise punishing environment. She alone encouraged the fantasies of future accomplishment that were Mother's most potent defense against parental rejection and abandonment.

The most traumatic abandonment occurred when Mother was about two, and the deeply unhappy Mary suffered a "nervous breakdown" (possibly a depression). Mother and her older sister and brother were sent to live with Nama for a year in California. Mother vaguely remembers that they took a train across the continent with Nama, feeling quite lost and bewildered. As kind as Nama was to them, the experience can only have been traumatic for all three children. Mother was too young to remember much of that visit, but she did recall that Nama had been very warm and comforting to her. Several years later, Nama came east to live with the family in Gananoque, and Mother was old enough then to spend hours enjoying her company, talking, and learning to sew. Here she basked in the desperately needed feeling of being loved. Nama's room in the family house remained in Mother's memory as "full of sunshine and the smell of lavender … I was cherished there …" When she was herself a grandmother, Mother wrote, "Where would that little girl have been without you, Nama?"

Mother always suspected that Mary was quite envious of her special relationship with Nama: "Grandmother loved me … and you never forgave me [that]. You took it out on me even though … since a two-year-old needed *something,* I had turned to her for love and support."

In the years immediately following her breakdown (from about 1906 to 1909), Mary took her children to live with her in Europe. Mother speculated later that Mary had been looking for something that marriage and Gananoque could not provide: a place where her beauty, energy, and talents might be appreciated and rewarded. When she was not able to find this panacea on one part of the European continent, she would pack up her children and move to another. Mother remembers attending numerous schools in which she did not know the language being spoken, and never being in one place long enough to learn the language before Mary would abruptly move them elsewhere. Mother later ascribed much of her extreme isolation as a child to those years of constant dislocation. She later wrote that she could not remember "one child met and liked and played with in all the years we were away."

There were, however, enjoyable moments of play with her siblings—for example, playing church on Sunday afternoons with Don as the preacher, mimicking their father's devout sermons. "Holding his hands with all the fingers curved and touching—just like Father," he would stand on a stool to preach, and "he didn't miss a single idiosyncrasy of the performance," Mother remembered with pride. Don's impudent sermons were cherished memories that she often shared with me as a child:

> Dearly beloved brethren, is it not a sin, for when you peel potatoes to throw away the skin? For the skin feeds the pigs, and the pigs feed you. Dearly beloved brethren, is this not true?

There must have been solace for all three siblings in these irreverent performances. And they were, as it turned out, a training ground for brother Don, who grew up to become an Episcopal priest like his father. But in spite of his more devout relationship to his parents and the church, Don was always an admiring supporter of Mother's rebelliousness—even in the darkest hours of her troubled relationship with Mary. Mother was deeply grateful to him, all her life, for this much-needed affirmation and love.

During these early years, there was only one strategy through which Mother seems to have connected directly with Mary, and that was as Mary's caretaker. Given the emotional pressure on my mother to become prematurely strong and independent, it is not surprising that she gradually came to experience Mary (with her perpetual unhappiness and her "nervous breakdown") as a very vulnerable person. In a piece headed "Trenton, 1912," Mother describes how Mary (then quite heavy) was injured after unwisely trying to join her children in a game of three steps across the curb:

> Well of course she fell kaplunk—disaster! No bones were broken but there were bruises, and her pride was severely injured. To bed she went and I elected myself nurse. Someone must stay awake with her all night, we figured. She said "yes," Sally should do it. I did, at least I tried, and felt special and big and needed.

Some twenty years later, when Mary was ill and required surgery, it was my mother who was summoned to care for her, though Mother was living in Europe at the time and her other siblings were much closer by. Mother had long been Mary's preferred caretaker, illustrating the complexity of Mary's feelings toward her daughter. She fought Mother's willfulness and considered her a "wicked" child; she envied Mother's rebellious spirit and independence; and she relied on Mother's great competence to support her emotionally and physically in her moments of greatest need. For Mother's part, she had become a caretaker par excellence as the only means of feeling important to Mary. Indeed, it was her exemplary skills as a caretaker that Mother relied on all her life as a means of affirming her importance to others.

Mary and the children went from Europe back to Gananoque just a year or so before the death of Mother's father in 1910. Because the children had been away from Gananoque for four years, they had spent very little of their young lives actually living with their father. And Mother, as the youngest child, hardly knew him at all. This contributed to her feeling, upon his death, that she had "lost what I never really ever had."

Within the next year, Mary moved to Trenton, New Jersey, and soon thereafter, the children were sent to boarding school. (Summers still seem to have been spent together in Gananoque.) Mother wrote one brief vignette about her life at St. Margaret's, a boarding school in Toronto, where she was, at age nine, the youngest child. Here, once again, she found herself "a black sheep—a bad egg," considered to be "naughty [and] fresh." She was not a terribly good student, but she sustained herself, as she always had, with fantasies that her special gifts would someday bring her fame and honor, exposing a pitiful lack of discernment on the part of teachers and school mistresses who had failed to appreciate her audacious intelligence.

Mother's first astonishing demonstration of ability and determination was her success in getting into college. She had not seemed to her high school teachers a likely candidate for higher education (especially given the small number of women who went on to college in the early 1920s), and she was actively discouraged from taking college preparatory courses. But she had spent many weekends alone in the school library while other students were away visiting their families, and she had become an avid reader. When the time came, she insisted on taking the college entrance exam, and (she later told me with understandable pride) she studied secretly at night in the bathroom down the hall from her dorm room (comfortably ensconced in the bathtub) because the bathroom light was always on. To everyone's amazement, she passed.

Mother completed a B.A. degree at Barnard College, an M.A. in sociology at the University of Pennsylvania, and began a doctorate in education at Columbia University. During these years, she discovered modern dance and was thrilled with the realization that her body was not only strong and capable but was also very beautiful and graceful. She began to envision a future for herself as a dancer and as an important innovator in dance education. Though she was never to fulfill this destiny, she continued to identify herself as a dancer throughout her life.

It was research for her doctoral dissertation on dance that took Mother back to Europe in the late 1920s to study the way dance was taught in Germany and Austria. While she was in Vienna in 1929, she met my father, and two life paths—at once both strikingly different and compellingly similar—crossed and joined together.

...

My father was born in Frankfurt, Germany, in 1902, and spent his first few years living with his mother in the nearby town of Buehl. His mother, Karla Abrahamsen, came from a wealthy Jewish family in Copenhagen. She had married a man named Valdemar Salomonsen a number of years before she became pregnant with my father, and the name Salomonsen appeared on my father's birth certificate to provide a semblance of legitimacy. But Valdemar had actually abandoned Karla within hours of the wedding, and was far away in North America when my father was conceived several years later. Although it is not technically accurate to say that Karla became pregnant "out of wedlock," it is true that she had never lived with her husband and that he could not have been the father of her child. To avoid a family disgrace, she was sent away from Copenhagen to have her baby, virtually alone, in Germany. And there she continued to live alone with my father after his birth.

When Dad was three years old, Karla married again—this time to the man (Theodor Homburger) who was my father's pediatrician. My father was told that Theodor was his real father, though he would certainly have been aware at the age of three that Theodor had not always been a part of his life. He later wrote:

> All through my earlier childhood, they kept secret from me the fact that my mother had been married previously; and that I was the son of a Dane who had abandoned her before my birth. They apparently thought that such secretiveness was not only workable (because children then were not held to know what they had not been told) but also advisable, so that I would feel thoroughly at home in their home. As children will do, I played in with this and more or less forgot the period before the age of three, when mother and I had lived alone.

How remarkable that forty years later, my father—now a child psychoanalyst—would try to deceive his own children, relying on the same naive assumption: that children do not know what they have not been told.

My father's own story then takes a startling turn. It seems he was in the Black Forest one day, at the age of eight, watching an old peasant woman milk a cow. She looked up at him and asked, "Do you know who your father is?" My father rushed home to his mother to demand an explanation, and she told him *part* of the truth: that Theodor was not his real father and that she had been previously married. She did not, however, clarify that her previous husband could not have been my father's biological father, since he had left Europe several years before my father's conception. My father did not grasp this fact until, as an adolescent, he began to glean the truth from relatives in Denmark. It is striking to me that in the passage quoted above, written when Dad was in his seventies, he *himself* obscures this crucial point. Even in his old age, it was still a source of shame to this celebrated man that he had been an illegitimate child.

After it had become clear to Dad that Salomonsen was not his biological father, Karla still refused to tell him the real identity of this all-important person. When directly confronted by my mother many years later (who wanted information about the genetic heritage of her own children), Karla still declined to answer. She claimed that she had promised her husband, Theodor, lifelong secrecy at the time of their marriage, and she wished to remain faithful to her commitment—despite the fact that Theodor had been dead for several years.

I have heard this story many times over the years and have always felt angry with my grandmother for what seems an incomprehensible lack of empathy with my father's need to identify his missing father. I struggle to respect her commitment to Theodor as well as the demands of her own pride, which was, after all, twice damaged. She had first married a man who proved a scoundrel and departed for America only a day or so after their wedding. Then, living in Denmark as an abandoned bride, she became pregnant by another man, who would not (or *could* not?) marry her. I can hardly imagine the shame that such a predicament must have caused her in 1902. Nevertheless, it is difficult for me to forget the years of anguish she caused my father by her unwillingness to help him with his deep feelings of loss regarding the missing figure in his life.

My father never did learn the identity of his father. Even Friedman's exhaustive investigation into this matter in the 1990s failed to provide an answer. Since there are no longer any surviving relatives in Denmark who experienced this scandal at first hand, it seems that the truth is lost to history.

What was clear to me, beginning in my childhood, was that my father suffered terribly from the sense that his real father had abandoned him and had never cared to know him. "Adoption was the great theme of Erikson's life," Dad's boyhood friend Peter Blos told Betty Lifton. "He talked about it all the time, speculated on the possibilities." And when Lifton asked Dad directly why he had not pursued the question of his paternity more vigorously, Dad replied, "If my father hadn't cared enough about me to want me then, why should I look him up now?" This reluctance to pursue the matter reflects, I think, the ultimate dread that his father might *still* refuse to know him, making the abandonment even more personally devastating than before. But his lifelong inhibition against pursuing the question of his parentage also reflected a need to protect his mother from a truth that was obviously too painful for her to reveal. And this was a self-sacrifice that cost him dearly in terms of his own emotional well-being. "The unnaturalness of not knowing your origins makes you feel unnatural," Betty Jean Lifton asserts. "There is the presumption that something is wrong because it can't be told. And when a child is raised with secrets, he feels his whole life to be wrong." My father suffered very much from a sense of having been unwanted by his biological father and of having been betrayed by his own mother in her failure to help him come to terms with this enormous loss.

The tone of my father's own written reflections on the topic seems to me to reveal how little he ever acknowledged to himself the depth of his anger toward his mother for denying him information about his real father, or toward his stepfather for making this deception a condition of their marriage:

> If the malignancy of the identity crisis is determined both by the defects in a person's early relationship to his mother and by the incompatibility or irrelevance of the values available in adolescence, I must say that I was fortunate in both respects. Even as I remember the mother of my early years as pervasively sad, I also visualize her as deeply involved in reading … and I could never doubt that her ambitions for me transcended the conventions which she, nevertheless, faithfully served.

And about his stepfather, he "was anything but the proverbial stepfather. He had given me his last name (which I have retained as a middle name) and expected me to become a doctor like himself."

He credits both parents with having ambitions for him, equating such ambitions with the kind of acceptance and support that would make a child feel genuinely cared for. He does not acknowledge that their narcissistic claims on him resulted in the neglect of his own deepest needs. Their respective agendas for him were radically different, but in each case, their expectations were shaped more by their own narcissistic concerns than by empathy with his emotional vulnerability as a traumatized little boy.

My father's mother had suffered humiliation and was, understandably, lonely and depressed in the years she lived alone with Dad. (He acknowledges her "pervasive sadness" in the quotation above.) She needed not only emotional comfort from him but also help in healing her narcissistic wounds. She perceived my father as a sensitive and gifted child and took pride in his obvious intelligence, sharing with him her own passion for philosophy and art. For him, this must have represented a lifesaving way to connect with a mother who was (for the first years of his life) sad and subdued, and who then shifted her primary allegiance abruptly to a new husband. She does not seem to have understood the extent of the trauma that her marriage to Theodor, and her subsequent deception of my father, caused him.

I don't believe Dad ever felt very secure in his mother's love. Though she clearly adored him, her narcissistic fragility—her deep preoccupation with her own wounded pride—prevented her from responding to Dad in a way that addressed *his* pain, *his* needs, or *his* reality. If Dad eagerly embraced her ambitions for him, accepting them as a measure of her love, it was his way of securing a connection with a mother who, in spite of her deep affection, withheld the emotional nourishment he needed most.

Karla's marriage to Theodor offered her an opportunity for social respectability after a period in her life when she had been essentially exiled from Danish middle-class society. She agreed to a radical change in lifestyle to meet Theodor's requirements. He was a very conventional man—a highly respected doctor and an Orthodox Jew. His image as a professional and as a leader in the Jewish community in Karlsruhe (where they lived together) was of the utmost importance to him. Though Karla's commitment to Judaism—and to social propriety—was far less rigid than her new husband's, she agreed to keep a kosher home and to play an active part in the activities of the liberal temple of which Theodor was a leading member. This was quite a dramatic departure from the bohemian lifestyle Karla had adopted during her years as a single mother in Buehl. There, my father later recalled, she read a great deal ("what I later found to have been such authors as Brandes, Kierkegaard, Emerson") and socialized primarily with artists. Some of these acquaintances, my father believed, were his first male role models. His lifelong identification with these early figures was covertly supported by his mother in vicarious fulfillment of her own abandoned fantasies of a freer, more bohemian existence. There is no doubt that she encouraged in Dad the very interests she had had to suppress in herself when she married Theodor. And this could only add to the strain between Dad and his very proper stepfather.

I am astounded at how little I know of Theodor, who was a central part of Dad's life for so many years. Although my grandmother (known affectionately as Muts to her children and grandchildren) loomed large in our awareness from childhood on, Dad rarely mentioned Theodor—neither to complain about him nor to express affection. I never heard Theodor described or quoted, and although his name was given to my brother Kai as a middle name, I was barely aware of the connection this represented with Dad's family history. I don't recall even being told about it when Theodor died, whereas Dad wept openly when he informed me of his mother's death. It was as though Theodor had barely existed for Dad, though I know that this cannot have been the case. The question is why someone of such importance in Dad's early life was relegated to obscurity in his adult years.

My parents had adopted the name Erikson (their own invention) soon after they arrived in the United States, giving Theodor's last name, Homburger, the status of a middle name for Dad. For many years this was as much as I knew about Theodor: that there were tensions in his relationship to Dad, and that Dad's name change was symbolic of the emotional distance between them.

Dad's half-sister Ruth describes Theodor as having been a caring father but not someone who was warm or demonstrative with his children. Being a man of his times, he worked very long hours and had little leisure time to be with his family. Nor did he talk with them. Ruth remembers that he hardly spoke a word as they walked together to temple on Friday evenings and Saturday mornings. And while Ruth never doubted Theodor's love for her, this absence of verbal communication can only have made my father's sense of connection with him the more tenuous.

The relationship between Dad and Theodor was, understandably, precarious from the start. There was good reason for my father to resent him, and there was good reason for him to resent my father. Dad once said to Betty Lifton that

> an adoptive father may unconsciously treat a son as not descended from him and therefore opposite of his own kind. The father can feel hostility because the son doesn't have his sense of humor or other traits. "Genes enter into it," [he] said, acknowledging the importance of genetics in creating closeness among family members.

There was much to arouse such feelings of hostility in Theodor, whether they were conscious or not. My father was physically quite different from him in appearance: blond and blue-eyed and, eventually, six feet tall; Theodor was dark-haired, brown-eyed, and of smaller stature. This difference, in itself, challenged any feeling of relatedness they might have developed. But it was not just his Scandinavian appearance that set Dad apart from his stepfather. Dad's earliest identification had been with his mother's intellectual and artistic nature, and with the artistic lifestyle of her friends. His emotional alliance with her and with her bohemian past also stood in the way of the identification with his stepfather that Theodor craved from him. While Theodor was a very disciplined and hardworking man, Dad was not a disciplined student and made no significant effort to be more like his stepfather in this respect. Dad was ambivalent in his commitment to Judaism and also resisted the idea of becoming a doctor (though later, of course, he did become a different kind of doctor, acknowledging Theodor's influence). Theodor must have felt personally rejected by him from the very beginning of their awkward relationship.

Dad experienced Theodor as more protective of his own social and professional image than he was of Dad's enormous vulnerability as a child needing love and personal affirmation. This is suggested in a reference Dad made to Theodor years later (1968) in a letter to my brother Jon. He states that Theodor "always got angry" when personal demands were made upon him by Dad or by his half-sisters Ellen and Ruth.

Of course, a European father in the early 1900s was not expected to be attuned to the psychological needs of his children or, indeed, to be much involved in their upbringing. So it is not surprising that even Theodor, a doctor of children, simply assumed that the child he rescued from illegitimacy and to whom he had given his good name would be grateful, would respect and mirror him and would behave in a way that affirmed his cherished beliefs and values. It is understandable that Theodor was not inclined to give Dad what he needed most, which was to have his own sense of differentness recognized and at least tolerated, if not affirmed. He needed help in developing a positive self-image that included those characteristics that set him apart from his stepfather and from the people around him. Because of his Scandinavian appearance, he was often "referred to as 'goy' "in his stepfather's temple; his schoolmates, nevertheless, taunted him for being a Jew. He suffered the isolation and shame of a misfit. And Theodor's persistent demand that he embrace Orthodox Judaism and the norms of bourgeois German-Jewish culture only enhanced Dad's sense of alienation from his stepfather.

Painfully aware of Theodor's disapproval of him, and contemptuous of Theodor's "bourgeois" values, Dad comforted himself with a rich fantasy life regarding his "real" parentage: "My sense of being 'different' took refuge (as it is apt to do even in children without such acute life problems) in fantasies of how I, the son of much better parents, had been altogether a foundling." (Dad's willingness to replace his mother along with his stepfather in these early childhood reveries reflects, I think, his deep sense of having been betrayed by Karla.)

Fantasies about the identity of his real father were still a vital part of Dad's emotional life well into his adulthood. As his children, we knew he imagined that his biological father had been a Dane of upper-class status, if not of royal blood. He believed this man was a Gentile and thus had been unable to marry Karla at the time of Dad's conception. Here, again, is the stuff that fairy tales are made of: Dad cherished the belief that he was the very special child of a Danish nobleman, whom he no doubt resembled in appearance and perhaps also in artistic and intellectual temperament. This fantasy ennobled his devastating childhood situation, providing an identification with someone socially superior to the conventional Jewish doctor whose affirmation and support Dad must have longed for, but whose requirements were impossible for him to meet. Dad's sense of failure in relation to Theodor clearly intensified his preoccupation with the noble Danish father of his reveries, and fueled his fantasies of one day demonstrating his secret connection with this superior being by becoming famous for the gifts inherited from him.

As it turned out, Dad's "imaginings" about his father may have only slightly exaggerated the truth—a truth that Dad's Danish relatives undoubtedly whispered about within his hearing when he was a child. After Karla's death in the 1960s, Dad received a letter from one of his Danish cousins, Edith Abrahamsen, providing the first real corroboration of his suspicions about his paternity. Referring to conversations with two other Danish cousins, Edith wrote:

> A few days ago I went to Svend's office and talked the matter over with him and I have also discussed it with Henny and they both agreed with me that we ought to tell you what we remember as having been told to us.... Henny says that she was told that your father was not a Jew.
>
> Svend['s] ... father had told him that your father was a highly intelligent man of a good Copenhagen family. In Svend's memory he was in some way connected with art. Henny has a similar idea.
>
> None of us know the name.

I still remember how profoundly Dad was affected by this letter, which he shared immediately with the family and with close friends. At the age of sixty-two, he was still desperately hungry for the vital information that had been withheld from him all his life.

By his late adolescence and early twenties, Dad had come to feel "intensely alienated from everything my bourgeois family stood for." He had graduated from the Karlsruhe gymnasium (roughly equivalent to American high school and junior college) at the age of eighteen, with mediocre grades at best. He briefly sought formal training as an artist, showing considerable talent, and soon adopted the tentative identity of a wandering artist, a bohemian lifestyle made possible, he acknowledged, by money his mother secretly made available to him. Theodor was, by now, openly intolerant of Dad's prolonged avoidance of social and financial responsibility and would not have looked kindly on Karla's continued efforts to help him.

Indeed, this period of Dad's life was more troubled than the romantic image of the wandering artist might suggest. He later wrote: "I will not describe the pathological side of my identity confusion," during that time, but "no doubt such disturbances assumed at times what some of us today would call a 'borderline' character—that is, the borderline between neurosis and adolescent psychosis." He was, by his own account, quite seriously disturbed, his functioning marginal at best. When he became convinced that he could never be a great painter (that his artistic talent would never win him wide acclaim), he abandoned his wanderings and returned to the home of his mother and stepfather, virtually immobilized by depression.

It is hard to say how this depression might have resolved itself if Dad had not been invited by his oldest friend, Peter Blos, to come to Vienna to help teach in a school created (by Dorothy Burlingham) specifically for children connected with the Freudian circle. Dad acknowledges that Blos "came to my rescue in my late twenties" (he was actually twenty-five) not only by securing a job for him, but also by arranging his trip to Vienna and helping him to learn to work regular hours, a difficult adjustment for my father. It was through Blos that Dad met both Anna and Sigmund Freud. Their recognition of Dad's extraordinary gifts, and their encouragement of him, was to change his life forever.

> It must be more obvious now what Freud came to mean to me, although, of course, I would not have had words for it at the time. Here was a mythical figure and, above all, a great doctor who had rebelled against the medical profession. Here also was a circle which admitted me to the kind of training that came as close to the role of a children's doctor as one could possibly come without going to medical school. What, in me, responded to this situation was, I think, some strong identification with my stepfather, the pediatrician, mixed with a search for my own mythical father.

Dad entered into an analysis with Anna Freud and began his own training as a psychoanalyst, a career in which his intellectual genius would soon be revealed to the world. But just as his identification with his stepfather (acknowledged above) took a radically altered form in his decision to become a child psychoanalyst, Dad's identification with Freud was soon to take a radically altered form as well—a form that was to acknowledge the interrelationship between intrapsychic phenomena (which was the focus of Freudian analysis) and the social, cultural, and historical contexts within which they occur. This theoretical shift brought Dad recognition as a great innovator in psychoanalysis, but also resulted in a painful rejection by his own analyst, Anna Freud, who perceived his work as a betrayal of Freudian theory. (Decades later, Ms. Freud was to say to Margaret Brenman-Gibson, "Oh, well, Margaret, Erik's work is not much. It was designed to make my father's work palatable to Harvard freshmen.")

A "habitual stepson," my father once wrote, might "use his talents to avoid belonging anywhere quite irreversibly." And so, indeed, this talented stepson did. His real psychoanalytic identity was not to become established until he had left the Freudian circle *and* had replaced his stepfather's surname with a name of his own invention. It was then, with my mother's collaboration, that he developed his own psychoanalytic perspective—a perspective that won him fame as Erik H. Erikson. It is almost impossible to imagine how his career might have unfolded without the emotional and intellectual support of my mother who—herself a rebellious spirit—nourished and encouraged his revolutionary brilliance.

From Homburger to Erikson

By my parents' account, it was concern for my older brother Kai that became the impetus for their eventually changing their last name from Homburger to Erikson.

As a small child transplanted from Austria to America, Kai was reportedly taunted by his schoolmates with the familiar American word "hamburger, hamburger." Wanting to relieve him of this embarrassment, Mom and Dad chose a last name for Kai in keeping with Scandinavian tradition: Kai, Erik's son, became Kai Erikson. Kai has no memory of having been teased about his name or consulted about a possible name change. It has always seemed to him that it was our parents' own preference, first and foremost, which motivated this decision.

And, of course, the name change had other unmistakable meanings for both my parents, since it signified my father's disassociation from his stepfather and suggested that he had, in effect, invented himself (Erik Erik's son). Indeed, it was my parents' view that they *had* invented themselves. After all, my mother had earlier changed her own first name from Sally to Joan, distancing herself from the family that had called her Sally and from her negative self-image as a child. So the adoption of a last name of her own choosing also signified the next step in *her* reinvention of herself. Nevertheless, whenever my parents were later asked for an explanation for this momentous decision, it was Kai's needs they cited as the determining factor.

I remember that the whole family went before a judge, a number of years later in California, to formalize the change.

Chapter 4

They Meet

My parents met in 1929 at a masked ball held at Maria Theresa's summer palace on the outskirts of Vienna. My father, then twenty-seven, was dressed as a young Turk, complete with fez. My mother, twenty-six, was dressed as a bejeweled dancer. I have no doubt that she looked stunning. The first invitation to dance must have been inspired primarily by the shape of her lovely face and body because for their first few dances together my parents were still masked. But even with his penetrating blue eyes partially concealed, Dad also struck Mom as a dashing figure. And when the two of them paused to reveal their faces, the mutual attraction was complete.

After hours of dancing, they walked to a nearby park and sat talking late into the night, recognizing each other—both consciously and on deeper levels of awareness—as fellow survivors of difficult beginnings. They confessed to each other their mutual sense of alienation from the conventional family life they had known as children: Episcopal in my mother's case and Orthodox Jewish in my father's. They revealed to each other a mutual desire to embrace a radically different way of life, less circumscribed by religious or social convention and more personally gratifying to them than the value systems they had rebelled against in their youth. And they confessed to each other the fantasies of great achievement that had been their refuge as isolated and unhappy children. Each glimpsed in the other a potential ally in the quest for liberation from the past—an ally who might provide the kind of love and support for which they both desperately hungered. Each also identified in the other personal resources that, combined with their own, could help them achieve the recognition they longed for. Not long after their meeting, they flouted the conventions of their respective family backgrounds by moving in together. Mother soon became pregnant with my older brother Kai.

It was almost uncanny the way my parents' early experiences had prepared them to connect with each other as adults: Dad had never known his biological father. Mother had hardly known hers. They had both experienced crushing parental disapproval and had felt estranged from their families and peers. Both had felt like misfits in the social worlds in which they had grown up.

Yet each of my parents had also been admired and championed by one all-important adult: Dad by his mother, Karla; and Mother by her grandmother, Nama. These affectionate and admiring relationships had made both of my parents feel

DOI: 10.4324/9781003645757-5

like special children, with idealized self-images that helped them cope with the feelings of rejection and disapproval that had plagued their childhoods.

Dad, of course, imagined himself the son of a Danish nobleman, socially superior to his parents and his peers. His grandiose fantasy life developed around the intellectual and artistic gifts that he believed he had inherited from his Danish father as well as from his mother. These were the gifts his mother cherished and that they both imagined might someday bring him special recognition. Perhaps these exceptional abilities also reminded his mother of the man who had fathered her child.

In Mother's case, it was her personal independence and self-reliance, her adventurous spirit, and her fearlessness as an explorer that her grandmother greatly admired in her, and that had made her feel special as a little girl. She had come to rely exclusively on her own personal resources in a parental environment that offered her so little nurturance or protection. She was especially proud of her strong and capable body and took meticulous care of it throughout her life. This trust in her own resources fueled a drive to nurture others less confident of themselves, or in need of emotional support and guidance. She was a healer.

Mother's own fantasy life revolved around the conviction that her strong body, acute intelligence, and bold spirit could carry her wherever she wanted to go in the world, and could conquer all adversity. Her mission was to embolden others by sharing with them her innate wisdom and supreme self-confidence. She had planned to make her mark as an innovator in dance education, believing this to be the medium through which she would communicate her intuitive understanding of the human body *and* the human spirit, and put to good use her remarkable healing energy.

It is significant that in the pursuit of their own heroic dreams, each of my parents fulfilled the denied ambitions of their mothers. We know that prior to Karla's marriage to Theodor, she had chosen for herself a bohemian lifestyle in which she was surrounded by artists and immersed herself in reading philosophy. Although she chose social conformity over the pursuit of her youthful interests, she clearly invested Dad with the task of fulfilling her own secret longings as an intellectual. Dad's attraction to the new and iconoclastic field of psychoanalysis seems to have reflected his mother's suppressed inclinations.

Mom's mother, Mary, seems to have been thwarted in all her efforts to find fulfillment in life—inhibited, it seems, by both a need for conformity and a pervasive fearfulness. Mary fought hard against Mother's rebellious spirit, but Mother always suspected that behind that disapproval was a secret envy of Mother's willingness to flout convention and to explore the world so fearlessly. Mary was afraid to go sailing with her children, for example, though Mother knew that she longed to do so. How she must have envied the courage Mother regularly displayed when she sailed off in her little dinghy.

Mother's mission to inspire and heal others seems to have had its origins in her response to the fearful and depressive Mary, whom Mother cared for when she was injured or ill, and in whom she must have longed to instill a greater feeling of self-confidence and enthusiasm for living.

It is striking that Mary had traveled through Europe with her children, looking, Mother suspected, for a place where her beauty, energy, and talents might be appreciated and rewarded. She returned from her travels disappointed and unfulfilled. It was Mother who traveled Europe twenty years later (sometimes alone on a bicycle) and found in Vienna exactly what Mary had longed for most: love *and* admiration.

My parents both had troubled mothers whom they longed to heal, which surely had some bearing on their mutual commitment to the healing arts. They both felt oppressed by their parents' anxious conformity to social convention and needed to affirm themselves by defying that convention. And, just as important, I believe, they had both relied heavily on a sense of being special—on grandiose fantasy—to help them cope in their early years. So their mission as healers was infused with a rebellious spirit and with an undeniable sense of grandiosity. They both wished to change the world.

Despite these similarities in their backgrounds and aspirations, my parents had developed very different personality styles and characteristic ways of relating. These differences were as important in defining their relationship as were the commonalities in their experience.

Dad had just emerged from a severe depression when he first met Mother, and he struggled with a depressive tendency all his life. His childhood experience of abandonment and rejection had left him plagued with self-doubt—not about his intellectual abilities, but about his more fundamental adequacy as a human being. In the intellectual realm, paradoxically, he possessed the monumental self-confidence and personal courage required to forge a new and brilliant path in psychoanalysis, but in the realm of intimate relationships, he felt deeply insecure and unsure of his footing. He craved constant support, guidance, and reassurance from others. And when that was not available—as during the period of his youthful wanderings through Europe—he became more and more emotionally unstable, until he could no longer function on his own, and returned home. Those years of wandering demonstrated how difficult it was for Dad to care for himself, physically or emotionally. His depression only lifted when his friend Peter Blos arranged for his trip to Vienna and provided (together with his analyst, Anna Freud) the necessary emotional sustenance and guidance to help him adapt there. But it was my mother who offered Dad the lifelong source of security—the emotional anchor—he needed to realize his full potential as a brilliant intellectual.

Dad's dependency needs and his struggle with self-doubt were not obvious to most observers once he had become established professionally. But his insecurity does seem to have been evident to one of his key informants among the Yuroks—a wise old woman named Fanny. Dad reports in *Childhood and Society* that Fanny laughed merrily at his uneasiness about interviewing her alone. "You big man now," she reassured him.

Dad's humble self-presentation and his perpetual quest for reassurance were generally experienced by others as charming in a man so brilliant and so successful. Fanny may have been attuned to Dad's genuine insecurity, but among those more impressed with his intellectual gifts, his style was interpreted as a sign of deep self-confidence. Only a very secure person, it was assumed, would be unembarrassed to reveal such vulnerability. And it is true that Dad's reliance on others for narcissistic supplies reflected a grandiose sense of entitlement to such support. His admiring mother had, after all, provided such affirmation when he was a child, and experience had since taught him that his openness in expressing his needs actually *enhanced* his charisma rather than detracted from it. (I'm sure it was an asset in his relationship with the perceptive Fanny as well.)

After Dad became famous, of course, it was considered a great honor to be called upon—as his surprised admirers often were—to give him advice and comfort. But his pursuit of reassurance was not simply the charming humility it was generally interpreted to be. It expressed a persistent and tormenting self-doubt.

In marked contrast to Dad's openness about his needs, Mother had learned early on to conceal hers. She had found it deeply humiliating to reveal her longings to her cold and withholding parents, and she had coped with emotional deprivation by denying her need to be taken care of. While Dad could openly express feelings of sadness or insecurity, and felt little shame in asking for support and nurturance, Mother hid her vulnerability behind a facade of almost complete self-sufficiency, supercompetence, and supercheerfulness. She was good at *everything* and seemed perpetually confident and high-spirited. She was delighted with the report that someone had once said of her, "That woman even enjoys brushing her teeth!" This was, indeed, the impression she gave.

And Mother *did* have an extraordinary capacity to enjoy life and to share her enjoyment with others. Her spontaneity and enthusiasm brightened the lives of countless friends and acquaintances. But her radiant exterior also concealed deep feelings of shame and inadequacy instilled in her by parents who thought her a difficult child—bad, mean, and selfish. And, of course, it concealed her grief and anger at having been so rejected.

Mother never felt as confident about being lovable as her social grace and ebullience suggested. In truth, she struggled with profound fears of abandonment. She related to others by helping them, giving to them, teaching them, *healing* them. She could only trust relationships in which she was the provider of resources greatly needed by the other. Her role as the caregiver had to be the dominant element in her relationships. Only then could she allow herself to be cared for in return. She was a very generous, thoughtful, and devoted friend, and she gratefully received much generosity and devotion from others. But it was essential that she always be the ultimate expert in the art of caregiving. This assuaged her fear of being perceived again, as she had been as a child, as a mean-spirited and selfish person. It also guaranteed her a sense of special importance to others. But it left her with lifelong feelings of anger and deprivation about her own dependency needs, which had been so thwarted when she was a child, making it difficult for her to express them effectively or to gratify them as an adult.

Mother had become the *giver* of care as a strategy for gaining acceptance from her unnurturing and disapproving mother. And it was the closest she could come to gratifying her own needs as an adult—by giving to others the exquisite caretaking she herself had longed for all her life.

Mother was most confident in circumstances in which she felt absolutely indispensable. Dad offered her a relationship in which her indispensability was obvious, and he rewarded her for her care with a childlike adoration and dependency. He revered her for her boldness of spirit, her striking self-confidence, her capacity to enjoy life, and her skillfulness in dealing with the practical world. His self-esteem was greatly enhanced by his connection with a woman whom he perceived to be so powerful. But just as deeply as he craved her support and reassurance, she craved his reliance on her. It was her covert need that her competence and self-assurance be easily visible in the relationship, highlighted by the enormity of his overt need for her. Only such a relationship could assure her of being important to the one she loved and could allay her fear of abandonment.

But, of course, it was not just Dad's dependency that felt deeply nourishing and healing to Mother; it was also his warmth and affection. They were both capable of loving tenderness and expressed their devotion to each other in a variety of ways—being physically as well as verbally affectionate with each other. Their mutual affection was also delightfully revealed in their sense of humor. They took great pleasure in their lifelong ability to make each other laugh.

And Dad enriched Mother's life through the depth of his intellect. She stood in awe of his intellectual gifts, which she seems to have recognized almost instantly upon their meeting. Although she had already earned an M.A. in sociology and was embarked on a Ph.D. relating to the teaching of dance, Mother was not as confident of her intellectual ability as she was of her boldness of spirit and her more artistic and pragmatic gifts. Her self-esteem was greatly enhanced by her association with this brilliant and promising young psychoanalyst, and she dedicated herself to providing the physical, emotional, and intellectual support he needed to maximize his enormous potential.

Mother was not the profound thinker or writer that Dad was, but she brought to their intellectual partnership her own passion for ideas relating to mental health—ideas that were eventually to win her great respect and admiration in her own right from the many people whose lives she touched. From the perspective of Dad's career, however, it was Mother's fearlessness in defying convention and her unflagging confidence in *his* ideas that provided the emotional and intellectual inspiration he needed to become a truly great innovator.

Clearly, Mother had longed for marriage and a family (she wasted no time getting pregnant with Kai, and my parents married soon after she realized he was on the way). Her relationship with Dad provided her with a way to have the family she desired as well as the vicarious rewards of outstanding achievement. She also acquired a position of considerable authority—not only in her personal relationship to Dad, who acquiesced to her in most matters other than the content of his work, but also as the practical head of a growing family, *and* as a dominant influence in the unfolding of Dad's extraordinary career. While Dad enjoyed the benefits of being taken care of, Mother enjoyed the security of her role as the indispensable caretaker as well as the power she exercised within the steadily widening sphere of Dad's fame.

Mother must have imagined that her own contribution to Dad's work, as his intellectual sounding board and editor (and much later as a coauthor), would eventually lead to her sharing more of his public recognition than she ever really did. She very quickly relinquished her plans for her own career. She never completed the dissertation research that had originally brought her to Vienna. Her ambitions for herself in modern dance were superseded by her ambitions for Dad—and for herself as a participant in his career. His work, and her part in it, became the new focus of her fantasies of achievement. This was a trade-off made by a great many ambitious women of Mom's generation who thought their talents were best invested in the support of a promising male star. But though she gave up her career in dance almost immediately after meeting Dad, she continued to identify herself as a dancer for the next seventy years.

My Parents and Psychoanalysis

My parents were both embraced by the circle around Freud in Vienna, and were appreciated for their respective gifts. They both taught in the small school (the Heitzing School) started by Peter Blos, where Mother was admired for her exceptional beauty, personal competence, and intelligence as well as for her qualities as a teacher. However, my father's personality and intellectual background made him far more receptive than my mother to the psychoanalytic theory being developed in this community. With her degrees in sociology and education, Mother was dubious from the start about the lack of attention to sociocultural factors in the narrow intrapsychic focus of Freudian psychoanalysis. She not only questioned the theory, she lacked respect for the clinicians who were beginning to make use of it. She had begun an analysis herself with a man by the name of Ludwig Jekels, and soon began to feel contempt for his efforts to analyze her. She told me years later how she had resisted his interest in her unconscious by fabricating dreams to report to him—dreams he accepted as authentic and earnestly interpreted to her. What Jekels did not know (and had no adequate chance to find out) was that Mother had survived her punishing childhood by being secretive about her most intimate thoughts and feelings. This pattern was so deeply embedded by the time she arrived in Vienna that not even *she* knew how profoundly it affected her way of relating. I don't believe she had any genuine interest in revealing herself to an analyst, but she went through the motions because it would have seemed strange *not* to in the social environment in which she found herself.

When Jekels suggested that Mother was developing an attachment to him, she almost laughed in his face. He was not a physically prepossessing man, she explained to me, and he was (in her perception) *old.* His suggestion that she might have feelings for him therefore struck her as absurd.

I don't know how much Jekels's own personality and analytic style may have been responsible for Mother's lack of engagement in this relationship, but her contempt for him says a great deal, I think, about her own fear of *becoming* attached to him—or of letting him come to know her more deeply. It was essential to the success of this relationship, after all, that *he* be the healer and that *she* be the emotionally more vulnerable one—an impossible balance for Mother to sustain. Soon after his reference to her possible feelings for him, she left her analysis.

It was only when (a decade later) she was overwhelmed with despair following the birth of Neil that Mother allowed herself to seek help from a psychoanalyst—overcoming, by sheer necessity, her terror of her own feelings of helplessness and dependency. This relationship lasted for the one week that Mother visited Frieda Fromm-Reichmann in Taos, New Mexico. It is significant, I think, that she did not consult any of the well-regarded psychoanalysts in the nearby San Francisco Bay Area from whom she might have gotten more extended help. It seems she needed to limit both the length of her dependency on the person she consulted and the depth to which her feelings could be explored.

When she was in her nineties, Mother confessed to Larry Friedman that she had "never acquired an abiding interest in psychoanalysis," nor had she ever really wanted to gain self-understanding through psychoanalytic exploration. I never knew her to recommend psychoanalysis *or* psychotherapy to anyone whose personal problems came to her attention, no matter how severe those problems might have seemed. Her advice was always of a more practical nature: perhaps a return to school, the development of a new artistic skill, or a change of career would provide what was needed to dispel confusion, depression, or anxiety and restore mental health. So it is rather remarkable that she allied herself with a budding psychoanalyst and spent her life straddling the line between his analytic perspective and her own more artistic and pragmatic approach to healing.

What made my mother an indispensable collaborator in Dad's work—despite her own doubts about the efficacy of psychoanalytic practice—was her implicit faith in *Dad's* ideas. She thought his work profoundly important and used her keen intelligence to facilitate the development of his unique style and point of view, despite the fact that her own intellectual style was quite different from his. In my parents' later years together, Mother wrote five of her own books, which reflected a range of nonpsychoanalytic interests and made it clear how different her style of thinking and writing was from Dad's: *The Universal Bead,* 1969; *Saint Francis and His Four Ladies,* 1970; *Activity, Recovery; Growth: The Communal Role of Planned Activities,* 1978; *Wisdom and the Senses: The Way of Creativity,* 1988; and *Legacies: Prometheus, Orpheus, Socrates,* 1993. Yet she was able to support his work with an intelligence and a passionate conviction that lent power and authority to his genius. The irony is that her contribution to the development of groundbreaking psychoanalytic theory was underlaid by a personal aversion to analytic self-exploration *and* by a profound skepticism about the value of the "talking cure."

Mother's paradoxical relationship to psychoanalysis was to express itself very clearly when my parents moved to Stockbridge in 1951 to work at the Austen Riggs Center. Mother created an activities program at Riggs that offered patients the opportunity to engage in a range of artistic pursuits. Her widely admired program broadened the treatment approach not only at Riggs but at many other mental health facilities that subsequently followed the Riggs example. In truth, however, Mother had more confidence in the healing potential of the arts than she had in the psychoanalytic work being done by the professional staff at Riggs. She fought against the intrusion of any analytic interpretation into the patient's art therapy. To the extent that the creative process revealed important unconscious material, it was creative expression itself that healed, making analytic interpretation quite unnecessary in her view.

Mother's pervasive doubts about the efficacy of psychoanalysis began to affect Dad's relationship to the field soon after their meeting. Although Dad was then deeply involved in the movement taking shape in Vienna, he was also a man who had characteristically "lived on the boundaries." He wrote much later that despite his excitement about what he was learning in Vienna, he had needed to "cultivate not-belonging and keep contact with the artist in me" so that his psychoanalytic identity could develop outside the confines of Freudian orthodoxy. What is clear in retrospect is that Mother's lack of enthusiasm for the work being done in the Freudian circle supported Dad's inclination to think independently and encouraged his own drive toward non-conformity.

Most specifically, Mother's skepticism reinforced Dad's ambivalence about his training analysis with Anna Freud. Here, too, Mother's personal needs intersected with an astute assessment concerning the shortcomings of the work being done.

Mother's personal need to be indispensable to Dad required that he rely exclusively on *her* for basic emotional sustenance. I believe this precluded Dad's full involvement in *any* analytic relationship once they had met. It even prevented Dad from maintaining his close friendship with Peter Blos, who was hurt and bewildered when Dad withdrew from him in Vienna after Mother had entered the picture. Dad and Peter had been close companions since their years together in the gymnasium in Karlsruhe, and they had played a major role in shaping each other's lives and ways of thinking. It was the crucial intervention by Peter that had brought Dad to Vienna in the first place—an intervention that Dad later acknowledged as having, effectively, saved his life. Nevertheless, the bond between these two friends suffered after Dad met Mother, and it was never fully restored—even after both men had immigrated to the United States with their families and had become renowned for their work in the same field. Peter suspected that it was Mother who was unable to tolerate their continued intimacy. Having seen the intense pleasure in Dad's face when he and Peter *did* meet from time to time, I am convinced that the loss of this relationship was costly for Dad as well as for Peter.

But Mother was also alarmed, understandably, that Anna Freud seemed a rather cold person who lacked empathy with Dad's yearning for information about his biological father. It seems that Ms. Freud dismissed Dad's fantasies about his missing father as a "family romance," encouraging him to give up his preoccupation with his biological roots and his desire to learn more about his father. Mother, to her credit, recognized the seriousness of this empathic failure. It increased her concern that Dad was not getting what he needed from his analysis. There is no doubt that Mother's feelings about Dad's relationship with Anna Freud played a significant part in Dad's decision to terminate his analysis before Ms. Freud felt it appropriate for him to do so.

Discussing this issue with Larry Friedman many years later, Mother said she had thought that Dad needed a male therapist to help him work through issues relating to his missing father. Yet following his termination with Anna Freud, she did not encourage him to seek further analysis with a man. If the basis for his ending with Ms. Freud was really a concern for the effectiveness of their work together, why didn't Dad seek out another analyst who could better help him to explore the issues that continued to haunt him?

Dad could not have committed himself to another relationship as intimate as an analysis, even with a man, once the partnership between my parents was established. And he never dared to explore his conflicts more deeply. Even in the crisis period following Neil's birth, when Dad struggled with intensely painful feelings (including his love for another woman), it was not a psychoanalyst he turned to for advice. It was a family friend—an *engineer*—with whom he shared his bewilderment. That seems astounding for a man who was himself a psychoanalyst and who had easy access to the most distinguished members of his profession. No doubt shame played a part in preventing him from revealing his predicament to someone in his own field. But it is also evident that he did not wish to explore his feelings or have them analyzed. He simply wanted advice about what to do. And in his choice of a confidant, he had also chosen the advice that he would inevitably receive.

From the start, my parents' relationship was based on a mutual commitment to avoid reflecting on the traumatic aspects of their childhoods and to heal themselves by achieving the extraordinary and attaining fame. Neither of my parents was inclined to explore the feelings of shame and inadequacy that were the residue of their early experience of rejection. It was their shared fantasy that they would, instead, rise above these depressive feelings through the achievement of stunning success and by winning the admiration of the world.

And as it turned out, my parents' relationship was perfectly suited to the realization of their heroic ambitions. My father did, indeed, become very famous. In addition, my charismatic parents succeeded in projecting an extremely compelling image of themselves and of their relationship onto the public screen. But there were personal costs inherent in the kind of relationship they had entered into in Vienna.

When my parents joined forces, they invested in each other in a way that helped each of them feel more personally complete and more capable of succeeding in the world. Dad vested in Mother the power to take physical and emotional care of him, to organize his life, and to negotiate the practical world for him. Mother vested in Dad the power to enrich her intellectual life and to enhance her status in the world through her association with his unique talent. As a result of this emotional—and literal—division of labor, each of them relinquished the opportunity to develop those qualities in themselves that they had vested in (or projected onto) the other.

In Mother's case, her belief in Dad's greater career potential diverted her from fully exploring her own creative potential. That might seem like a relatively small price to pay given the monumental success of the partnership into which she entered. But being partner to the great man was never as fully gratifying to her as she had hoped it would be. And if she was such a vital part of *his* success, what might she have accomplished on her own, following her own creative path and developing *her* talents fully? She would never know the answer to that question, but it haunted her. As great as were the vicarious rewards of Dad's fame, Mother always craved more personal recognition, not only for her part in his work, but also for the books she wrote on her own. Several of these found an appreciative audience, but none were received with anything like the acclaim that greeted my father's work. In this sense, Mother's own accomplishments, as impressive as they were, were eclipsed by the enormity of Dad's success, and I believe this was demoralizing to her.

Mother was adored and admired by a remarkable number of friends and acquaintances. But she lived with the knowledge that her own importance to others was infused, inescapably, with the aura of the great man she had married. The brilliance of the spotlight on *him* illuminated her as well, but this was, inevitably, a mixed blessing. She felt diminished by her dependency on this vicarious source of illumination. And she could not help but wonder how much of the adulation she received from others was the result of her own personal charisma and how much was the reflected glow of my father's celebrity.

Furthermore, Mother's role in the relationship meant that she would never receive the caretaking from her husband that she longed for, despite her difficulty in accepting care from others. For Dad to have focused on *her* needs would have required a sea change for both of them. It was a behavior unfamiliar to him and fraught with conflict for her. I think that the pronounced division of labor in their relationship, never examined by either of them, contributed to Dad's lifelong feelings of personal inadequacy and to Mother's lifelong feelings of personal deprivation.

Inevitably, it was a source of ongoing tension in their relationship. Dad expressed his resentment toward Mother's control through passive resistance in relation to practical tasks. For him to set the table involved countless questions regarding her preferences for particular plates, glasses, and so forth. Getting him out of the house to go somewhere was often a Herculean task, even after she had selected and laid out the clothes she thought he should wear. Mother lived in a state of palpable irritation (sometimes more controlled than others) with Dad's perpetual uncertainty about how to complete the simplest chores.

Nevertheless, Dad sustained the role of emotional dependent in relation to Mother, relying on his belief in her powers as a substitute for developing a greater sense of self-reliance. Her need to be indispensable to him through the decades of their life together actually discouraged him from ever becoming more autonomous.

And, of course, Dad knew (however conscious this overwhelming realization may ever have been) that an essential element in his relationship with Mother was his potential to be a star. Both brought fantasies of greatness to their meeting at

Maria Theresa's summer palace, but it was Dad's genius that was to be the vehicle for their joint ascension. Just as he had felt that it was his intellectual ability that fulfilled his mother's narcissistic needs and secured her love, it was clear that his wife, too, counted on his gifts to help fulfill her own narcissistic strivings. For all the care and devotion Dad received from both women, he would never feel loved just for who he was.

In truth, both of my parents were profoundly dependent on the achievement of fame and an idealized public image of themselves as a couple. It was the overwhelming need to feel admired by others that left them so vulnerable to the crisis posed by Neil's birth. On the one hand, the demands of caring for a disabled child were inconsistent with the aspirations to which they were desperately committed. On the other hand, the decision *not* to care for Neil was painfully incongruous with their ideal view of themselves. It especially contradicted Mother's self-image as a quintessential caretaker and healer, but *both* of my parents needed desperately to feel like loving and caring adults—more passionately committed to the well-being of their children than their parents had been to caring for them. And so they could not "own" their decision to institutionalize their disabled child. Dad deferred to the experts and did what he was told. Mother relied on the myth that the decision had been made *for* her—that she had been robbed of a voice in the matter. Had the conflict over Neil's care not evoked such early feelings of shame and inadequacy in both of them, the decision might have been worked through somewhat more successfully—not that it would have been an easy call for any couple under any circumstances. But a more mutual and rational process of decision making might have alleviated the self-torment that followed Neil's birth, the sense my parents shared of having done something unspeakably monstrous—so unspeakable that they could not acknowledge it to their own children or to anyone who was not directly involved in the event, and did not *have* to know. (After the publication of Lawrence Friedman's 1999 biography, in which the story of Neil was revealed, several of my parents' closest friends acknowledged to me they had known nothing of Neil's existence.)

My parents' relationship was constructed on a pattern of emotional avoidance that cost them dearly in the course of their lives together. Most obviously, their inability to talk about painful emotional issues limited the amount of intimacy they could share with each other or with their children, and left them terribly vulnerable to the inevitable tragedies of life. Whether they were *unwilling* or *unable* to deal more directly with the emotional damage of their childhood years, this avoidance of unhealed wounds prevented resolution of the deepest problems that afflicted them and created a distance among all the members of the family while my brothers and I were young and not yet able to break the pattern of silence that had been imposed upon us.

On the surface, my parents' life together was blessed and serenely happy, and sustaining this image was of paramount importance to both of them. They shared an ability to rise above even devastating personal problems and feelings (as they had done so often in the Orinda years) to make a public appearance consistent with their idealized image as a couple. Of course, they *did* share a great deal of genuine love and pleasure in each other's company. They *did* have a long and deeply rewarding connection with each other. But their aura as a couple was also infused with the charisma of their respective personalities, which obscured (for most who observed them) the very human underside of their relationship: the resentments they felt toward each other and their mutual difficulty communicating about some of the most central issues in their life together and our life as a family.

Could it have been otherwise? Could either or both of my parents have benefited more from psychoanalysis? Could more direct attention to their emotional health and well-being—individually or as a couple—have significantly enhanced their relationship with each other? And if so, would that have contributed to, or detracted from, the enormity of their mutual achievement? I have no idea. I can only suggest the paradoxical relationship between my parents' idealized image as a couple and the actual limits of the intimacy they were able to share. It was my intimate experience of these two charismatic people that first led me to question whether there is, *by nature,* a paradoxical relationship between any larger-than-life public image—such as that of my parents—and the life-sized human beings who have generated it.

Chapter 5

Achieving the Fantasy

Fame

From Orinda to Stockbridge

When I was thirteen, my parents' fantasies of achievement began to be realized with the publication of *Childhood and Society* (1950). Soon thereafter, we left the house on Haciendas Road and moved to Stockbridge, Massachusetts. Kai was by then away at college, so he no longer lived in the family home. Jon still had one year of high school to complete, and he chose to stay in California so that he could graduate with his close friends. Mom, Dad, and I drove across the country with my cousin Ellen (daughter of my father's half-sister Ruth).

We stopped for a few days in Santa Fe, New Mexico, where Mother took me for a drive through the sagebrush and told me, for the first time, the truth about Neil—that, in fact, he had not died at birth but was still alive and doing reasonably well in an institution in California. In those days, a child with Down syndrome was still referred to as (offensive as it sounds today) a Mongolian idiot. And I remember so clearly how Mom ended the story, saying, with tears streaming down her cheeks, "That's why I never use the word *idiot* and never think it's funny when anybody else uses it."

I experienced the shock of confronting something I had sensed for many years but had, at the same time, been forbidden to know. I asked Mother a few questions about what Neil was like and what had happened, but she seemed overwhelmed by grief, and it was obviously very difficult for her to talk about it. I didn't need to ask why she hadn't told me before. Mother had never been able to talk about things that were too painful for her. And now the timing of her confession was crystal clear. We were leaving Neil behind, and that was the way it was supposed to be, emotionally as well as geographically. It was too late for fantasies about visiting him. I was not to entertain that thought—then or ever. And I never did.

We were moving away from the family life I had known in Orinda, leaving Kai and Jon on the West Coast as we drove east. And now I learned that things had not been as they seemed during those Orinda years. I would have to revise my view of the most central features of my family life: my parents who, I learned, would send a child away and then pretend he didn't exist and would keep such a secret from me; my own role as the youngest and most disabled child in this otherwise exemplary

DOI: 10.4324/9781003645757-6

family; and the family unit as a whole, previously consisting of five members—and now six. (To this day, I experience a moment of confusion when I'm asked, "How many siblings do you have?") This was a formidable task to carry alone into my adolescent years.

I was particularly alone in my struggle to make sense out of the past because, in their move to Stockbridge, my parents seemed to push the tragedy of Neil as far out of their conscious awareness as possible—focusing now on their new surroundings, new friends and colleagues, new tasks, and especially, on my father's new-found fame. *Childhood and Society* having just been published, my parents were received in Stockbridge as intellectual royalty, and they thrived on the celebrity.

Stockbridge and Celebrity

It was 1951 when my father joined the staff of the Austen Riggs Center, in Stockbridge, where he was revered by colleagues who were themselves well known in the field of psychoanalysis. Praise for *Childhood and Society* poured in from all over the country, and my parents embraced a new and deeply gratifying image of themselves as intellectual celebrities and social visionaries. Still, they did not surround themselves with the accoutrements of fame, or with others who were equally successful or well known. They continued to live as simply and modestly as they had before (albeit with more financial comfort and security) and maintained relationships with many friends who were not celebrated or renowned. These were the relationships in which they seemed most comfortable. Nonetheless, Dad's achievement had become the very cornerstone of his and Mother's sense of well-being and feeling of self-worth. Dad's success permeated every aspect of their life together, defining them in their relationship to each other, to their children, and to their many friends and acquaintances.

Understandably gratified by the tremendous response to his groundbreaking first book, Dad began to take on a new social persona. Though always an impressive figure, he had previously been a fleeting presence at most social gatherings, uncomfortable when the conversation was not intellectually stimulating for him, and restless when he was not at work. As a result, family friends had thought of him as charismatic but somewhat distant and aloof. Now, however, he became the undisputed center of attention at most of the social events he and my mother attended, and he enjoyed his celebrity enormously. His new confidence in the power and importance of his ideas greatly enhanced his aura.

Dad's very intimate writing style (widely acclaimed in the reviews of *Childhood and Society*) had made him seem to his readers like someone both brilliant in his subtle understanding of human behavior, *and* emotionally accessible and compassionate. In a social setting, people now gathered around him hoping not only for a kernel of great wisdom but also for the sort of intimate exchange that his writing seemed to promise. They were excited just to be near him and became oddly childlike in his presence—animated, deferential, and transparent in their eagerness to gain his approval. Even adults of considerable achievement in their own right seemed awed by him. In this environment, Dad himself became more completely alive and more emotionally responsive than I had ever seen him before—excited, in turn, by all the intense interest shown in him. I was witness to a highly charged dance between human beings eager to idealize a godlike figure and a man brought fully to life by their adoration.

To experience this phenomenon at close range is to understand the magical relationship between the charismatic world leaders who have shaped human history and their awe-inspired followers. My father was a heroic figure on a vastly smaller scale, and yet he now seemed to exercise such power over those who knew him and his work. Even to this day, I am startled by the awe on people's faces when they first discover my connection to him. Often they stare at me, dumbfounded, and ask, "Really?" Your father was *Erik Erikson?* And sometimes, "Can I touch you?" reflecting the magic associated with his image. It would be difficult to overestimate the excitement evoked in members of our species by proximity to a famous person—or even to a *relative* of that person. What is sometimes less obvious to the observer is the reciprocal excitement evoked in the celebrity himself when he is receiving the adoration of his public. I had never seen Dad enjoy himself so much.

Despite Dad's new level of confidence in his intellectual gifts, he had not changed much in the private domain. He was as plagued by self-doubt as ever, leaning on Mom and others for constant guidance and moral support. It is not that this insecurity was concealed in his public persona. Rather, it was experienced by Dad's admirers as an utterly charming humility—a delightful affectation in a man so successful and so secure that he felt no need to hide his vulnerability. Far from suggesting any genuine lack of confidence in himself, this self-effacing style only added to his charisma.

I remember these years as a golden era in my parents' lives. My father's fame was still new, giving it all the excitement of childhood fantasies magically fulfilled, and providing my parents with enormous satisfaction and enjoyment. If celebrity did not erase the suffering of the preceding years, it helped my parents to distance themselves from the shame and tragedy of Neil.

Mother shared in Dad's celebrity with an evident sense of entitlement. She had, after all, played an indispensable part in bringing his genius to the fore and in helping to develop his writing style. And, of course, she had always had a powerful charisma of her own. But her self-confident manner was now infused with the pride of extraordinary achievement and the aura of Dad's fame. Thriving on his celebrity, Mother began a major midlife transition of her own. In California, she had devoted herself to motherhood, home building, gardening and crafts, and playing a background (although vital) role as the editor of Dad's ground-breaking book. Now she craved a more visible professional identity for herself; so when she was given the opportunity to build an activities program for the patients at Austen Riggs, she threw herself into the assignment as vigorously as she had pursued her more personal projects in Orinda. She soon began to be recognized for her own enormous talent as the creator of a unique arts and crafts program for psychiatric patients.

In her late forties when she arrived in Stockbridge, Mother had many friends younger than herself whom she inspired, supported, taught, and guided with great generosity, but also with an uncompromising sense of certainty about what she believed was best for them. Rarely, to my knowledge, was her judgment questioned by those whose lives it influenced. Her wisdom was received as gospel, and it generated not only undying gratitude but often a deep reverence for her as a person. This was a source of profound difficulty for me because other people's eager acceptance of her guidance suggested that she was, indeed, divinely inspired and her judgment beyond question, even when her decisions in relation to *me* ran contrary to my most cherished wishes and desires. It was very difficult to stand up against my mother's convictions about what was best for me: about the way I should wear my hair, the way I should dress, or the way I should carry myself. She was often disapproving of my innovations, even when my friends thought them quite attractive. And always, in the end, I would bow to her judgment.

Nevertheless, I thrived in Stockbridge for the first year we were there, partly, I'm sure, because of my parents' new sense of well-being. I attended a boarding school located a few miles outside of town (The Stockbridge School) and blossomed there. Living at the school during the week gave me independence from my parents without making me feel isolated from them. I was thirteen and had grown taller and slimmer, making me feel more attractive. My new height gave me a particularly surprising advantage on the basketball court, where I found myself (it's still like a dream these many years later) the star of the girls' basketball team. I will always remember hearing my name yelled from the stands when we played against teams from neighboring schools, and I was counted upon to lead us to victory. I was popular for the first time in my life, and it was *exhilarating.* In spite of the shock of having so recently learned the truth about Neil, I (like my parents) began to recover from the emotional desperation of our life in Orinda.

But my own reprieve was to be short-lived. My parents decided during that year that I would be better educated at The Putney School, a boarding school in Vermont, two hundred miles away. Kai had attended Putney a few years earlier and loved it. I know my parents wanted me to have the same excellent educational opportunity they had made available to him, and Putney was, indeed, a more prestigious institution than the newly created Stockbridge School.

I had never trusted my own feelings as a legitimate basis for questioning Mother's supremely confident decisions, but I was grief stricken at the thought of leaving my new home *and* the school where I felt so happy for the first time in my life. Mother suggested that my popularity at The Stockbridge School was not authentic, but was, instead, the result of my father's fame. She thought that at Putney this might not be such a "problem." I was not aware that my high school friends knew much of anything about my father, and I did not *want* a more prestigious school for myself. I was comfortable at an institution with a lesser reputation, one that was less intimidating to me and closer to home. I was ashamed to tell them how much I still needed to have them nearby at the age of fourteen.

But I sensed at the time (and understand now) that Mother really needed to give herself over to the important professional opportunity that the Austen Riggs Center offered her. Perhaps she felt that parenting would be incompatible with the heavy demands of her new career. And perhaps I was an unavoidable reminder of the troubles my parents had so gratefully left behind with the move east.

And there was the undeniable reality, obvious to me only in hindsight, that as I moved into adolescence, my approaching womanhood and my popularity at The Stockbridge School were threatening to Mother. As beautiful as she still was in her late forties, it must have been difficult for her to watch as I enjoyed the kind of heady adolescent awakening— and especially the popularity with boys—that had been denied her in her own youth. Her early teenage years had been spent in a boarding school for girls, where she was not very well liked, and it cannot have been easy for her to watch as I became the center of this new kind of attention—nor did it help matters that Dad noticed and was appreciative of the changes taking place in my appearance.

For all these reasons, my emergence as a young woman would have to take place somewhere farther from home. My enrollment at Putney was not a matter for discussion. I did not dare express my intense feelings of despair and rejection, and Mom and Dad chose not to acknowledge what I did not tell them in so many words.

And so that September, Mom and Dad drove me to the beautiful Putney School in Vermont. I attended an orientation session and looked for them afterward to tell them what I had learned—trying to be optimistic and prepared to be very brave when it came time for good-byes. I was shocked to learn that my parents had already left for home, without saying good-bye. Mother later explained to me that she and Dad thought their unannounced departure would make the separation easier for *me*! In truth, I think it was *they* who were unable to deal with their feelings about this separation and were, therefore, afraid of mine. They must have been aware of the sense of abandonment their decision about Putney evoked in me, and this was simply too painful for them to address.

The overwhelming feeling of having been sent away, and the shock of their abrupt departure, intensified my own identification with Neil, who had been sent away without good-byes so many years before, and who had then been erased from memory. Knowing the truth about Neil, I was now more than ever aware of my parents' desperate need to avoid feelings of guilt, shame, or sadness. And fearful of being even further ostracized from their lives, I determined to conceal from them, as much as humanly possible, the feelings of rejection that now overwhelmed me and that cast a dark shadow over my years at Putney.

Looking back on those painful years, I cannot be sure how conscious I was at the time of my powerful identification with Neil and my overwhelming fear of suffering a fate similar to his. The depth of this psychological connection only became clear to me in retrospect when I began psychotherapy some fifteen years later and reported a mysterious dream to my analyst in which I had the facial features of a Mongolian. It was my analyst who gently reminded me of the other "Mongolian" in my family (who had been exiled, in my unconscious mind, to the nearby region of Siberia), opening up a wellspring of intense feelings and associations that would take years of analytic work to fully explore.

But during the years I was at Putney, I was more baffled than ever by the juxtaposition of my parents' need to avoid painful feelings and the powerful image of them as a couple that had now been embraced by the rest of the world. Everyone seemed to view them as quintessential parent figures—exceptionally wise and knowing and comfortable with the most sensitive of interpersonal issues. Everyone admired their wisdom and deftness at handling the emotional problems of *others.* I had no help with unraveling this mystery. No one else could help me to understand the relationship between my parents' impressive strengths and their human frailties because no one else seemed to *perceive* their frailties—or even acknowledge that they really *were* human beings. I don't remember anyone even hinting to me in the course of my adolescence that my parents were less than perfect.

I realize now that the adults who were most closely involved with my parents during this time seemed to me more like siblings than like my parents' peers. *Everyone* looked to them as parent figures and seemed desperate to have their love and approval. So I was one of a multitude who vied for their affection, and my own position in this legion was not at all favorable. I no longer lived at home, whereas some of my most serious competitors were part of my parents' everyday lives. I heard frequent stories from Mother about their creative lifestyles, their sublime artistic gifts, and especially about the generous things she had done for them and the devotion they showed her in return. The unavoidable truth was that I was ambivalent toward my parents in a way my myriad siblings were not. And my parents needed the unwavering adoration they got from these friends and admirers to sustain their sense of emotional well-being. My more complicated (albeit deep and genuine) love was not sufficient to reassure and nourish them in the way that the passionate devotion of others could. Understandably, it was those who adored them most enthusiastically who evoked from them the most effusive expressions of reciprocal pleasure and affection.

Nevertheless, Mom and Dad were warm and welcoming when I returned from school for vacations. I never complained about my loneliness at Putney or how out of place I felt there. I was deeply humiliated by my failure to thrive at the school they admired so much, and where my brother Kai's heroic reputation still hung in the air. This could only confirm my childhood conviction that there was something terribly wrong with me. I needed, above all, to pretend that this was not so and to conceal the shameful truth from Mom and Dad. For their part, my parents seemed completely oblivious to my difficulties in faraway Vermont.

Occasionally, Dad and I went for ritual lunches at the Morgan House in Lenox, which I enjoyed very much. But I was careful not to say anything about my general state of unhappiness. It was Dad who sought *my* reassurance, on these occasions, about issues relating to his professional life.

Mother would take me shopping for clothes, including one glorious weekend in New York, where we stayed at the Barbizon Plaza. On that occasion, she bought me a powder-blue coat, which remains in my memory as the most beautiful coat I have ever had—a symbol of the perfect gift Mother was so often able to give, and the pleasure it gave both of us. I wore it the next day when we walked together in the Easter Parade. Mother wrote, years later, about this enchanted moment: "Sue and I stroll down 5th Ave. There's spice in the air, it's spring. We've bought for her a long blue coat, the color of her vergiss-mai-nicht [forget-me-not] eyes. She has grown inches and walks a dance—'Gosh, Mom!' she says—" But after this heavenly weekend, I returned to Putney, where the dress code called for rugged outdoor wear and not for powder-blue coats. I kept this treasured gift from my mother in the back of my dorm room closet and tried it on secretly from time to time.

During these years, and for many years to come, my relationship with my parents was untroubled on the surface. There was never any question about the highest priority in their lives, which was Dad's career, and his still-growing fame. This, in addition to Mother's own success in her related work at Austen Riggs, is what sustained, nourished, and preoccupied them. They were affectionate parents, and I was an affectionate daughter. They seemed to enjoy my visits home and spoke of "showing me off" to their friends. When they were not working, we did things together, visited people, and laughed at long-standing family jokes. They were often very kind, supportive, and generous with me. It was clear to me how much they *wanted* to be good parents—and how warmly they expressed their love in the only ways possible for them.

But the relationship continued to be circumscribed by a requirement so pervasive that I was rarely even conscious of its power over me: it was essential that I *never* say or do anything, or express any feeling, that even hinted that they were *not* the ideal parents they so desperately wanted to be. My role was to support the image—now projected on a very large public screen—of the quintessentially good parents that both Mom and Dad had come to represent to the rest of the world. My complete discretion was required in public situations, of course, and also when we were alone together. It was not just avoidance of any reference to Neil (who was still alive at that time in a California institution). It was essential that I never express anger toward my parents or reveal to them my own unhappiness. Any suggestion of a grievance on my part caused them such distress that my own feelings faded instantly into relative unimportance. It was not until twenty years later that I confided to them how miserable I had been at Putney. And even this belated news so shocked and devastated them that I regretted ever mentioning it. As always, I moved quickly to reassure and to protect them from the implication that they had ever failed me as parents.

The memory of Neil's exile hung always over my careful relationship with Mom and Dad. Neil's birth and existence had caused them such shame and guilt that they banished him from awareness. I, too, experienced their pained withdrawal when something I said or did threatened their fragile sense of themselves. On some level, I always feared the possibility of excommunication.

Although I dared not be openly rebellious, my anger toward my parents did reveal itself in one way that stands out clearly in my memory: it was my lack of enthusiasm for Dad's success. I felt a strange (and, it seemed to me, unaccountable) resistance to reading his books; and as their numbers grew, I sometimes joked publicly about not knowing which one was which. I remember a large dinner party with family friends when I was asked whether I had read *Childhood and Society.* I responded coyly, "Isn't that the yellow one?" (a reference to the bright yellow jacket on the original hardcover edition). The joke was appreciated by everyone present, but I'm sure the message was not lost on my father: those books had gotten a lot more of his attention than I had, and I was not crazy about them.

One of my most striking expressions of disenchantment with the illustrious Erikson image occurred a number of years later when I graduated from Oberlin College, and McGeorge Bundy, then a dean at Harvard University, was the keynote speaker at the graduation ceremony. It happened that Dr. Bundy had recently hired my father to teach at Harvard, and so it was natural enough that my roommate and I should have dinner with him and my parents at the Oberlin Inn the night before the graduation. During the evening, Dr. Bundy asked me about my career plans, and I remember the fleeting sense of defiance I felt at telling him that I intended to become a secretary (which was, indeed, my plan). I don't remember my parents' reaction. They had never made an issue of my lack of ambition, but they must still have been taken aback by my deliberate use of the word *secretary* in this setting. It seemed that my only way of expressing resentment at my parents' obsession with achievement was to devalue what they valued most.

The cost of my careful compliance with my parents' needs—my efforts to protect their idealized image—during my high school, college, and early adult years was the suppression of so many of my own feelings and desires that I was an enigma to myself and to others, and I continued to lack all sense of personal ambition. I enjoyed college far more than high school, but continued into young adult life to be crippled by a lack of emotional separation from the monumental image of my parents. It wasn't until I reached my early thirties that I began to acknowledge the stultifying effect that my father's fame and my mother's indomitable will continued to have on me, and it was then that I devoted myself to the effort to understand my relationship with the giant figures who had loomed so large over me, holding me captive with their fragility as much as with their formidable strengths and gifts.

Chapter 6

Berkeley in the 1960s

I graduated from Oberlin in 1959 and set off for Berkeley, California, to begin my career as a secretary. My parents were still in Stockbridge at the time, but would shortly move to Cambridge, where Dad was to become a professor at Harvard University. My decision to start my adult life in Berkeley was a move away from my parents in a geographical sense, but certainly not in a psychological one. I was returning to the town in which I had spent my earliest childhood years, and I associated my parents with almost every aspect of the life on which I was about to embark.

It happened that my brother Jon was living in Berkeley at that time, and the five-year difference in our ages that had seemed such a huge chasm when we were children now dwindled into relative insignificance. This was when Jon and I bonded more than we ever had before. But though we talked about our earlier family life and about Neil, it never occurred to either of us to visit our mysterious brother, institutionalized less than a hundred miles away in Santa Rosa. Our parents' denial of Neil's existence had banished any thoughts we might have had about going to see him, and we never did. That made it all the more of a shock when Neil died in 1965, and our parents asked us to arrange for the burial of his ashes. (He had already been cremated in accordance with Mom and Dad's long-standing instructions to the institution that had cared for him.)

By sheer coincidence, Mom and Dad, who were in Italy at the time, had been having dinner with two of their oldest friends from California, Mart and Tom Proctor, when the call came from Kai relaying the news that Neil had died. Years later Mart described the evening to me in this way:

> The phone rang and Mom answered it, speaking in hushed tones. It was clear that she was shaken by the news she was receiving. She stayed on the phone for a few minutes and then spoke privately to Dad before the two of them returned to the dinner table. Mom informed the Proctors very calmly that the call had been from Kai and that Neil had died. The Proctors expressed their condolences. Although the Proctors were among the very few of my parents' friends who knew that Neil existed, and the circumstances of his institutionalization, my parents did not speak of Neil again for the rest of that evening. Mart was dumbfounded.

DOI: 10.4324/9781003645757-7

The next day Mom and Dad called Jon and me, asking us to arrange for the burial. (Kai lived on the East Coast.) They did not plan to return to the United States for a ceremony. Jon and I selected a cemetery we thought attractive in a nearby town; and as we discussed the burial arrangements with the cemetery staff, we were embarrassed to reveal that we knew nothing about the brother we were laying to rest.

"You are the brother and sister of the deceased?"

"Yes"

"You indicate here that you want his ashes placed in the children's cemetery?"

"Yes"

"But you also indicate that he was twenty-one years old at the time of death."

"Yes …, but we believe he was very … childlike."

"You believe …?"

"Yes. That's what we understand."

"I see … [trying not to look too puzzled]. Well, of course we can bury him in the children's cemetery if that's what you'd prefer."

Were we right that Neil was more childlike than adult at the time of his death? We realized that we had no idea. Imagining the anguish it would cause our parents if we opened up such questions, we never thought to do so—not before and not after the end of Neil's life.

We watched as Neil's urn was placed in the ground, feeling this must surely be a dream. We spoke to him and to each other of our sadness that he had been excluded from our family life, acknowledging that we could not be sure we would have wanted him to come live with us back in 1944, even if we had known that he was alive. How could we know that? But we *were* sure about the ongoing guilt and sorrow we felt toward the brother we had never been permitted to know or to love.

Love, Marriage, and a Secretarial Career

When I first arrived in Berkeley in 1959, I prepared myself for the career on which I was about to embark by attending secretarial school. I then took a job at the University of California in a research institute located only doors away from the research center where my father had worked when the family lived in Berkeley. Like a homing pigeon, I had returned to the world of my earliest memories—the world of my parents as I had first known them.

It was just a year or so before I met and fell in love with a graduate student at the university—an intellectual, of course; it could not have been otherwise. I was following in my mother's footsteps by becoming the supportive partner of a thinker and writer.

Harley and I were married in 1961. My parents had gone to Southern France for a year to give Dad an opportunity to write, and I had agreed before I'd even met Harley that I would join them in April of 1961 to type up Dad's handwritten manuscript. When Harley and I decided earlier that year that we wanted to marry, I wrote to my parents suggesting that Harley might join us in France at the end of the academic year so that we could be married there and travel in Europe on our honeymoon. Mom and Dad were thrilled and wrote me a joyful letter in support of this plan. The following story evokes some of my most loving memories of Mom and Dad:

> I went to France in April 1961—to the lovely hill town of Aspremont, above Nice—and typed the manuscript Dad had been writing. When Harley arrived in June, Mom and Dad drove me to the airport in Nice, and as soon as the flight had landed, they left me to greet Harley alone and spend the night with him in a lovely hotel not far from the airport. They knew how much it would mean to us to have time to ourselves before the family introductions began. When they arrived in Nice the next day to meet their prospective son-in-law, they could not have been more welcoming.

And that was not all. Mom had rented an enchanting hillside cottage that was to be available to the two of us immediately upon Harley's arrival. No need to wait for wedding vows to be exchanged. They had, after all, lived together in Vienna for some time before they took their own vows.

The wedding dinner stands out in my memory as one of those wondrous occasions that Mother, particularly, knew how to create. My brothers having arrived for the big event, the family gathered on the terrace of a restaurant overlooking the Var Valley—everyone happy to be there and in high spirits. Harley had been accepted into the family with a warmth that touched me deeply. When the moon rose, its soft light reflected in the Var River below, we were all transfixed by the beauty of the place and the perfection of the moment. It was a fairy-tale wedding in the Erikson tradition, but for once *I* felt like a central character in the fairy tale.

Our married life, however, was to take place in the real world. I was consumed with anxiety when we returned to Berkeley. I had graduated to the role of wife, and was now expected to fulfill that role with all the unwavering confidence and expertise that Mother had exhibited back in the early days of *her* marriage. I was entirely unprepared for the job, and developed several phobias that tormented me daily.

The 1960s were the time when my father's fame and popularity were at their peak. He was celebrated at Harvard as well as by the rest of the world. In the tumult of that decade, his understanding of adolescence and the "identity crisis" was captivating to Harvard students, who flocked (by the hundreds) to his classes. Harley and I both felt the burden of Dad's enormous celebrity as we fought for survival in the highly competitive academic world of Berkeley. Harley struggled to complete the requirements for a Ph.D. I worked as a secretary and also typed and edited his papers. I was compelled to play my mother's role as my husband's helpmate and "helped" Harley *far* more than he needed—imposing my own work inhibitions and compulsive perfectionism on his creativity in a way that was destructive for both of us and deadening to our marriage.

Harley's writing style was very different from mine. He was able to allow a multiplicity of thoughts to flow onto the paper more freely than was possible for me. And when I undertook to edit his work, I was overwhelmed by the sheer number of ideas offered on any one page. In my own need to bring order to this abundance, I sometimes deleted material that I could not bring sufficiently under control. Harley protested the surgery, but found it difficult to resist my organizational drive. So the richness of his writing was sometimes sacrificed to neater packaging.

We loved each other and had many happy times together when we were away from the world of work. But issues of ambition and career tortured us. Harley was (at that time) very much like my father in his vulnerability to self-doubt. I don't know how our marriage might have evolved if I had been more like my mother in being able to support my husband's obvious gifts with assurance, inner conviction, and especially with the drive my mother brought to the role of helpmate. But I didn't have that inner conviction; and unlike her, I was deeply ambivalent about the project at hand.

There was, first of all, the virtual impossibility that *anyone* I chose to marry could measure up to my family's Olympian standard of success. No matter how well I succeeded in the family tradition of helping him to become a "star," he would never be a star of the magnitude of my own father. So I felt trapped forever in a position inferior to that of my parents (and, I might add, to that of my brother Kai, who was soon to join the faculty at Yale). Harley had never aspired to such lofty heights, having grown up in a family environment less pervaded by grandiose ambition than mine. He wanted a university teaching position, but not on the grand scale that Eriksons tended to take for granted. He never imagined himself in competition with my father, nor was he as overwhelmed as I was by my father's fame. I think, in fact, that he enjoyed my parents (as they enjoyed him) and could have been content with the excitement that their celebrity sometimes brought into our lives. He had no idea, I'm afraid, how complicated my enmeshed relationship with my parents and my deep-seated ambivalence toward achievement would make our life together. But I suffered terribly from the fear that my life was going to be a pale imitation of my parents' magical journey.

It was not only my father's fame that made my own situation seem to me so impoverished. It was the illustrious image of my parents' life together that had been drummed into my awareness since I was a small child. I have referred to the stories my parents loved to tell of their earlier lives (both before and after their meeting in Vienna) that depicted them as characters in a beautiful fairy tale. These accounts enchanted their listeners and lent undeniable magic to my parents' image as a couple. But they left me feeling inherently and irrevocably inferior.

There were accounts of Mother's brave and defiant adventures as a child and her triumph over those who had failed to recognize her gifts (omitting any mention of Mother's devastating relationship with her own disapproving mother). There was the lingering fantasy that *just perhaps* my father's abandoning father had been part of the Danish royal family, and the seductive image of Dad as a gifted young artist, wandering through Europe in search of himself (omitting mention of his descent into depression toward the end of his romantic *Wanderschaft*).

There was the breathtakingly romantic story of my parents' meeting at the masked ball and Mother's equally enthralling account of their reunion the next day, when she ran headlong down the hill toward her rendezvous with Dad, afraid she would be late, and ran straight into his out-stretched arms. There was the charming story of their marriage on April Fools' Day, and of their life together in a rustic little cottage on a hillside in Vienna, where Mother did all the cooking and cleaning without benefit of running water, and from which she slid down a snow-covered hill on a laundry board to get to the hospital in time for Kai's arrival. I was so steeped in these romantic tales that when Harley and I passed through Vienna on our honeymoon, I was overwhelmed with nostalgia for *my parents'* early married life.

And, of course, there were tales of their brief encounters with the great Sigmund Freud, whom Dad glimpsed occasionally in the waiting room of the office Freud shared with his daughter Anna (Dad's analyst). How often did I hear it told that Freud had once said of my artistically gifted father, "He can help us to make them see" (that is, help the world to appreciate the aesthetic richness of psychoanalytic thinking). How often did I hear of Anna Freud's spontaneous reference to my mother as *die schöne* (the beautiful one)? It was as though these gods of psychoanalysis had smiled upon my parents, just as the supernatural forces in the fairy tale smile upon the hero and heroine, recognizing their specialness and lending support to their eventual victory over those who have persecuted them or failed to appreciate their gifts.

In fact, these stories had all the essential characteristics of the classic European fairy tale, which "depicts over and over an upward development [of the hero and heroine], the overcoming of mortal dangers and seemingly insoluble problems," in a courageous struggle that leads, inexorably, toward royal marriage and ascension to the throne. These reminiscences recounted my parents' rise from lonely childhood to a magical meeting with one another, and joint ascension to the modern equivalent of royal status: *fame.*

The frequent retelling of such tales conveyed my parents' own sense of having been chosen by the gods—a fairy-tale perspective that affirmed their special status in the world. And even knowing as intimately as I did the more emotionally troubled and complicated reality that lay behind the beautiful images, I was still susceptible to their magic. It made me feel that Harley and I were merely bystanders in my parents' charmed life rather than the central figures in our own life.

At the same time, I had grown up in a family environment pervaded by the emotional underside of the fairy tale of my parents' life together. I had experienced my parents as deeply wounded by early parental rejection. I had lived through the anguish of Neil's birth and banishment not only from our family life but also from our very *awareness.* I knew how emotionally fragile my parents were—how fearful and avoidant of central issues in their lives—despite their achievement of success.

I knew that fame had not brought them the peace of mind it promised—that they never stopped working or striving, always in pursuit of something more than they had already gotten. In fact, celebrity seemed to have made it more difficult for them to confront the deepest sources of their pain and self-doubt, actually compounding their need to remain hidden in ways that imprisoned them emotionally.

I was aware of all the ways in which fame had *not* healed my parents' wounds at the same time that I was overawed by the enormity of their gifts and accomplishments and felt irrevocably eclipsed by them. I could not dismiss the assumption so deeply rooted not only in my parents' psyches but also in the culture as a whole that fame represents the pinnacle of human achievement, and *must,* therefore, be the truest source of self-esteem and happiness.

How could I trust my own experience when it contradicted the passionate beliefs of so many others who never questioned the near perfection they attributed to my parents as individuals and to their life together as a couple? Even the people who knew my parents most intimately (besides my brothers and me) believed them to be as supremely contented with their lives and with each other as their image suggested and as one would expect such a glamorous couple to be. And those very few who had more direct knowledge of the issues that plagued my parents' life together never allowed this insight to threaten the idealization they held dear.

So I was profoundly conflicted about what I wanted in life, and only vaguely aware that this conflict was the source of my deepest unhappiness. I was, on the one hand, driven to try to replicate my parents way of being in any way possible—to share in their glory, in some small way, through mere imitation. But on a less conscious level, I was also terrified of being like them—addicted to achievement and to a glorified image that left the real sources of personal pain unattended and prevented the kind of genuine intimacy I had longed for all my life. I didn't really want to play the game the way my parents had played it, but neither could I imagine a meaningful alternative.

And there was yet another source of paralysis. In compulsively imitating my mother's role as helpmate to my husband, I was avoiding a deeply buried desire to have my own career, to focus on my own work rather than on someone else's. This reflected, I suspect, a powerful identification with my father and his way of thinking about things. But it was also a reaction to my mother's obvious disappointment that her role in Dad's work did not win her more widespread recognition in the scholarly world. I knew that being the helpmate was, on some level, a thankless job. But there were enormous emotional obstacles to my acknowledging my own desire for a career as an intellectual. On the one hand, it did not seem to me that my parents had ever considered me career material (as they had my brother Kai), since they had accepted my early lack of ambition without apparent concern. I was convinced that they did not think me especially capable. And I could think of nothing more humiliating than to reveal my intellectual limitations to the world. So it was much safer to stand behind the front lines—to be a good secretary and to serve as helpmate to my husband—than to expose myself to comparison with my world-famous father.

On the other hand (of course), I harbored secret fantasies of my own potential greatness—an inevitable defense against the feelings of inadequacy that plagued me. I was, after all, an Erikson, for whom nothing should be impossible. What if *I* were the ugly duckling in my own family story, and emerged a brilliant swan? I cannot describe the longing and the terror that such fantasies evoked in me. How could I even begin to put my talent to the test when greatness was the only acceptable standard of success? Or even worse, what if I *did* have success of my own? The children of addicted parents hate the substance that has dominated and depleted their family life; but they are also especially susceptible to addiction themselves, and often to the very same substance that has seduced their parents away from them. Though I was not conscious of it at the time, I was terrified of the potential for my own addiction to achievement. I feared that any success of my own would trigger a longing in me for the commodity that had obsessed my parents. And should that happen, I would become, like them, a prisoner to ambition, doomed to the loneliness of my childhood. The intensity of this conflict prevented me from acknowledging any ambition at all.

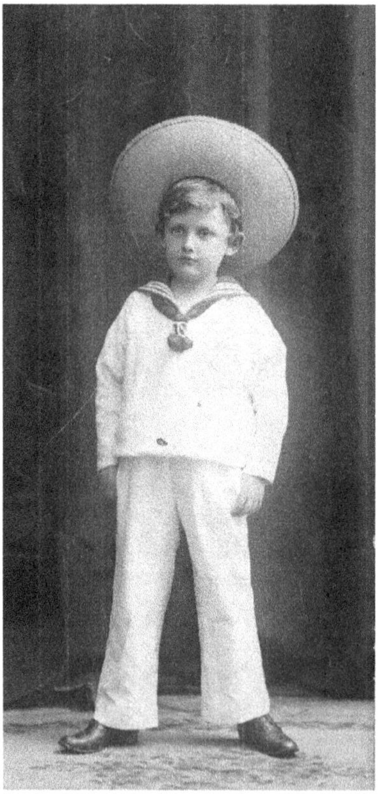

Dad in a sailor suit at about the age of five.

(Olga Klinkowstrom)

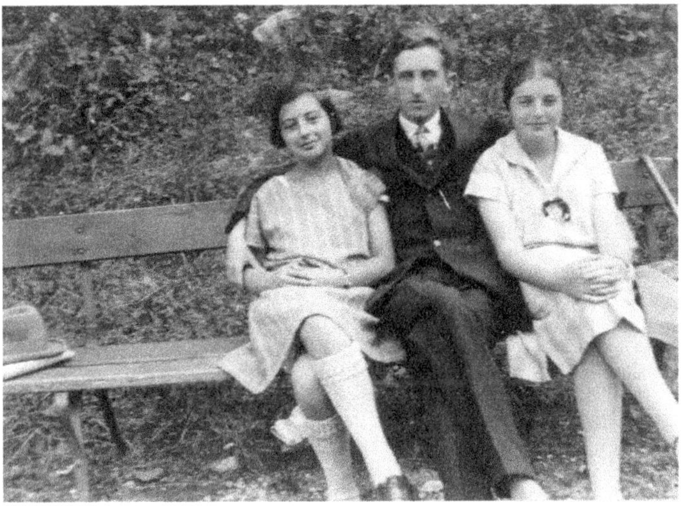

Dad with his half-sisters Ellen (*left*) and Ruth (*right*) in Karlsruhe in 1925. This was the period of Dad's deepest depression, which shows, I think, in his face.

(Photographer unknown)

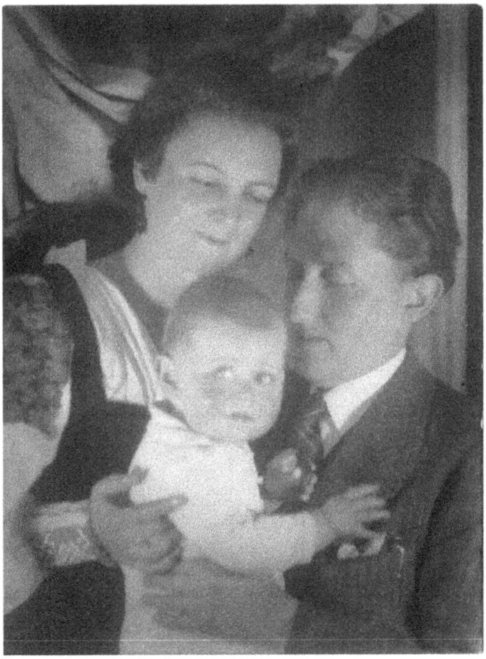

Mom, Dad, and Kai in Vienna in 1931. Here, Dad begins to look more like my father as I knew him.

(Photographer unknown)

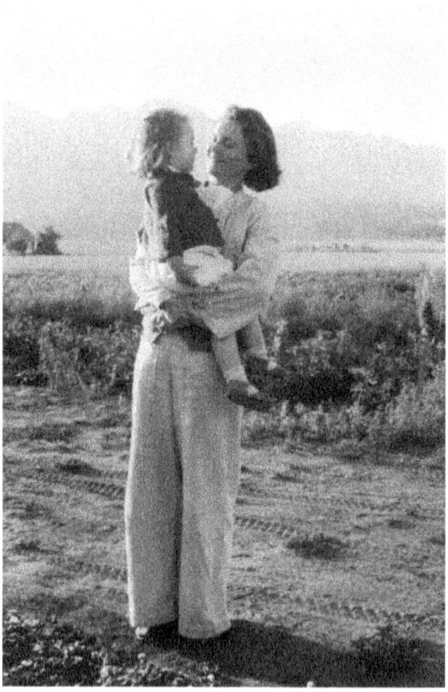

Mom and me in 1941.
(Carol Baldwin)

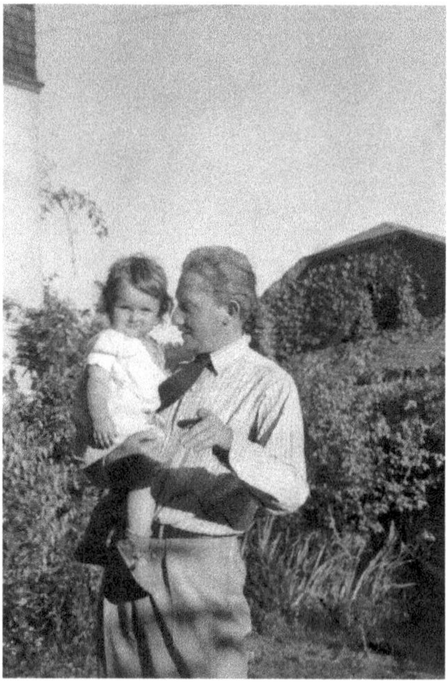

Dad and me in Berkeley, California, 1939.
(Photographer unknown)

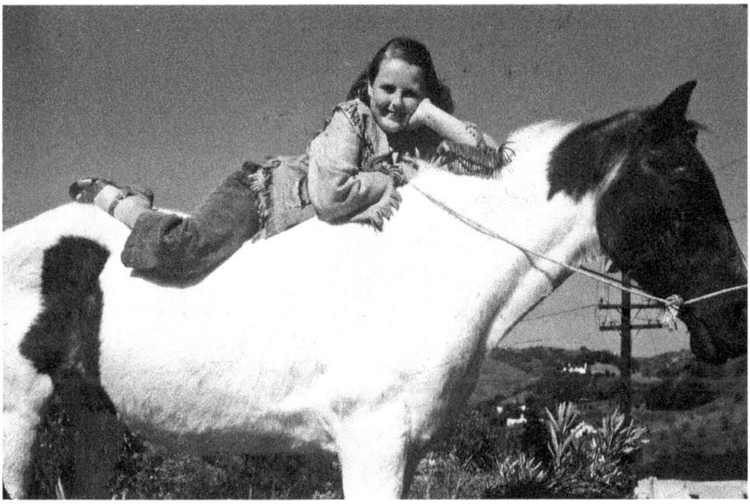

Me on my horse, Spot, where I was always happiest, circa 1948.
(Carol Baldwin)

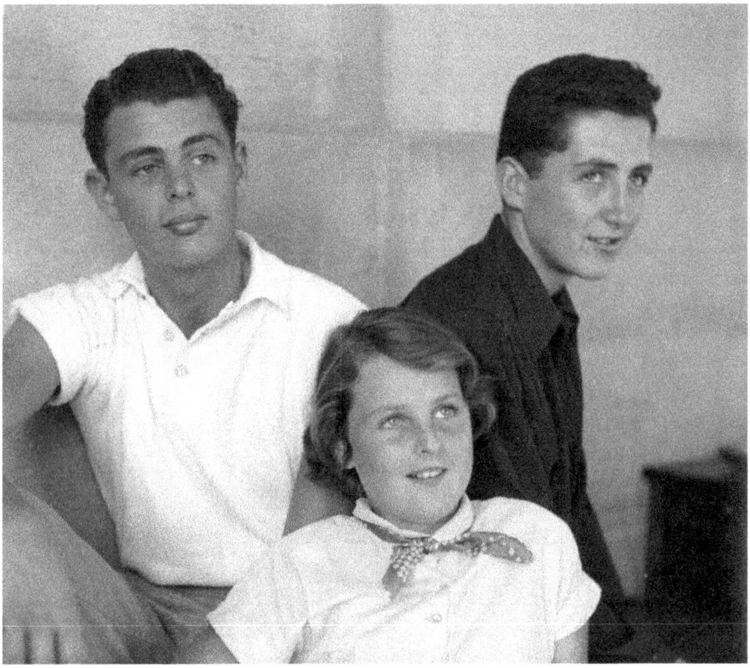

Kai, Jon, and me, circa 1949.
(Carol Baldwin)

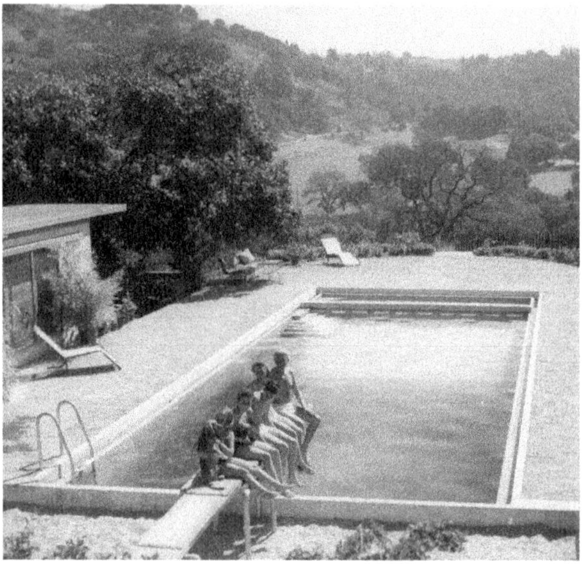

Dad, Mom, Kai, Jon, me, and my dog, Sandy, circa 1945. This was the idyllic setting and family image of the Orinda years.

(Carol Baldwin)

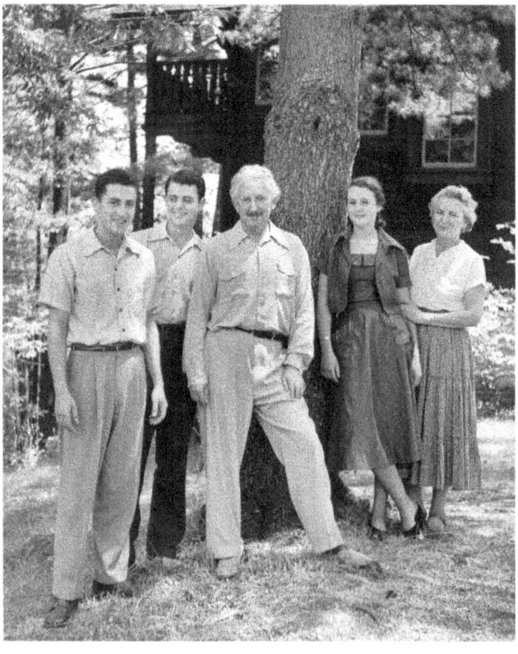

Jon, Kai, Dad, me, and Mom in Stockbridge in 1953.

(Clemens Kaiischer)

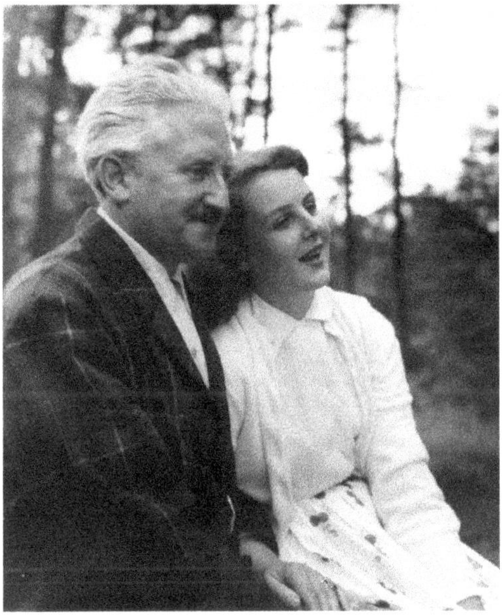

Dad and me in Stockbridge in the mid-1950s.
(Carol Baldwin)

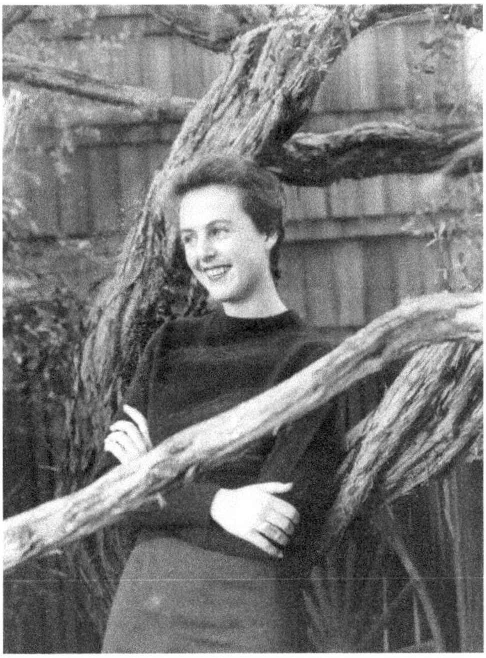

Me in Berkeley in 1960, just after I graduated from college.
(Carol Baldwin)

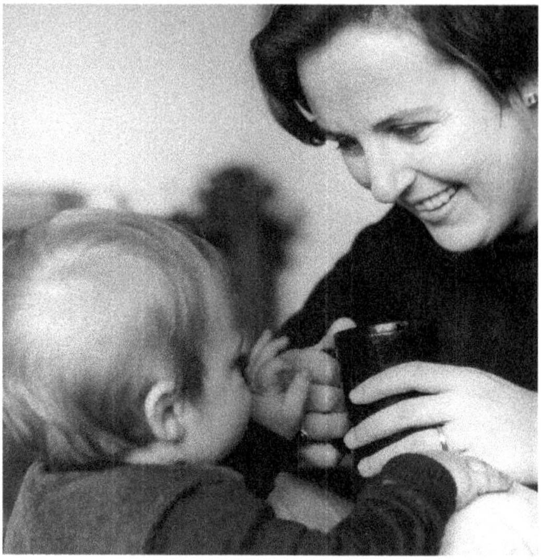

Per and me in New York City, 1970.
(Carol Baldwin)

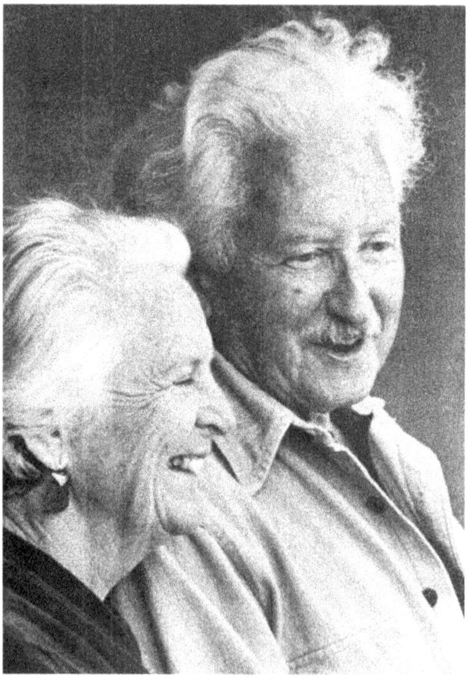

My parents in Belvedere, California, in the 1950s.
(Jon Erikson)

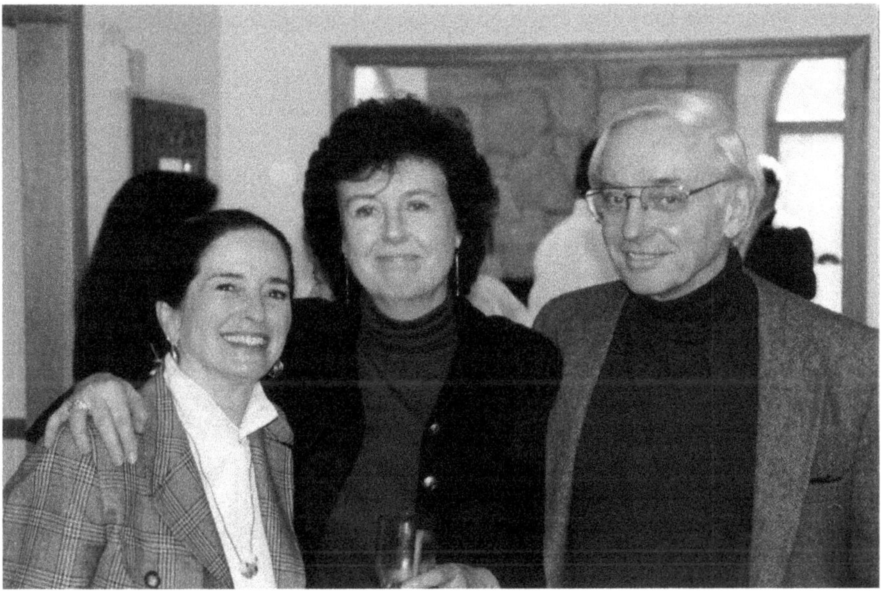

My cousin Ellen (daughter of my fathers half sister Ruth), me, and Bob at a birthday party for Ellen in 1998.

(Alex Greene)

I flirted with disaster during the eleven years of my married life by taking graduate courses in the social sciences (first anthropology and then sociology) and relishing them. I earned exemplary grades, but worked *so* hard on each and every writing assignment that I was convinced it was inordinate effort that had gotten me by rather than innate ability. I lived in anguish at the end of every semester—unsure that my efforts had been sufficient—until I received that life-affirming grade of A. Then, for a few days or even weeks, my grandiose fantasies flourished once again. But by the time a new semester had begun, I had resuccumbed to self-doubt. I could not risk getting an advanced degree, which would have been a *real* test of my scholarly ability. Nor did I dare to open Pandora's box to my deeply buried ambition. And so, despite enough credits to earn me more than one graduate degree, I never completed any formal program of study.

On the surface, it seemed that my life with Harley was progressing exactly as it should. He had dedicated himself to a field of study, the sociology of higher education, that truly fascinated him (and still does). He completed his Ph.D. and accepted a teaching position at New York University. I was excited but extremely anxious about moving to New York City, imagining that I would now have to dress like the women in *Vogue* magazine, a style to which I was *entirely* unaccustomed. I was relieved to find that Greenwich Village, the location of NYU, was not so very different from the Berkeley environment we had just left, and a whole new wardrobe would not be required.

...

Our son Per was born in New York in 1969. He was a beautiful baby—alert from early on and keenly interested in the world around him. We adored him and we seemed to have gotten where we wanted to go.

But as thrilled as we both were to have a son, my feelings of inadequacy as a mother only compounded my difficulty separating from the parents who still loomed so large on my horizon. I had imagined that giving birth to a child would establish me, at last, as a full-fledged adult. But I was totally inexperienced in the handling of infants, and I was—once again—up against my mother's confident expertise in this area (as in all areas, it seemed, of womanhood). She came to New York to help me care for Per during the first week after his birth, bringing calm and certainty and a blissful love of infants to bear on all the tasks at hand. Watching her attend to and soothe this tiny baby was like watching a beautiful ballet. And when she left for home again, I felt that a colossal error had been made in the organization of the universe: this precious child was left in *my* inadequate care, while the caretaker par excellence drove away to attend to other matters. It was several years before I could put that feeling in historical perspective: Mother had *always* made me feel that she was the supreme caretaker and could, if she were not so busy, make everything perfect for me; but she had more important matters to attend to, so I was left to care for myself as best I could. In Orinda, I had handled that sense of abandonment by riding horseback through the hills, taking comfort in the companionship of the powerful animal that responded to all my wishes and needed only the simplest care. Now I would have to muddle through on my own once again, without a horse to empower me.

The Turning Point

At this stage in Mother's own life, she was living in a small cottage in Vienna and teaching school, where she nursed Kai during recess. I lived in much greater physical comfort in a New York City apartment and had no job, but the combined tasks of caring for a small baby and supporting my husband's career were still overwhelming me. I was lonely and depressed, having had little time to make friends in New York before Per was born, and having few people to talk to about the endless mysteries of infant care. Once again, my level of anxiety (now about my competence as a mother) interfered with my ability to provide the psychological support that Harley needed as he embarked on his first academic job.

Harley and I had no experience in working through the kinds of problems that had beset our relationship from the beginning, and we had no idea what to do about the distance that was growing between us. It is painful for me to think back to that time, knowing what I do now about the necessity for communication between two people who long to be close to each other but have been driven apart by emotional forces they do not understand. We had no idea how to communicate with each other about the most difficult issues. We just grieved for the intimacy we had once shared. And we focused our attention on Per, showing him more love than we were able to show to each other.

I began to escape into fantasy during this time. I lived for my favorite TV shows (the *Upstairs Downstairs* series most of all). And when I began taking graduate courses, again in sociology, I imagined myself madly in love with one of my professors. I would stay up late at night, after Harley and Per were both asleep, weeping in sadness and longing. I could not imagine separating from Harley, but I knew something had to change. The conflict was agonizing.

It was in a sociology course at the New School for Social Research that I made a new and life-altering friend by the name of Virginia Reed. Our conversations were different from any I had ever had in my life. Virginia had struggled with difficult emotional issues of her own and had been helped enormously by psychotherapy. She talked openly and honestly about her feelings and experiences in a way that dazzled me from the start; and unaccustomed as I was to such candid self-revelation, I found it remarkably easy to tell her what I had never told anyone before: that I was deeply unhappy. Her empathy and optimism were a revelation to me. Virginia was about to end her work with an analyst who had helped her a great deal, and she suggested I meet with him. Because of the way she talked about herself and her therapy, I knew immediately that whatever had helped her to become who she was, *that* was what I wanted for myself.

But it was not easy to take that first step. Therapy was for me the forbidden fruit. I had envied my father's patients for as long as I could remember, imagining all they were able to tell him about their problems without his wincing in pain or withdrawing from them. In fact, Dad himself enjoyed telling the story of the psychoanalyst's daughter who, when asked what she wanted to be when she grew up, answered, "A patient." How deeply I had always identified with that little girl! Yet it had not occurred to me to seek help from psychoanalysis because it was not something that Eriksons *did.* Eriksons espoused psychoanalysis (or at least my father did), but they didn't become *patients.* They lived on the other side of the great divide between healers and those seeking to be healed. I was raised among healers and had tried my best to be a caretaker to my husband and child, but I felt hopelessly unsuccessful at it and now longed to defect. It was Virginia who helped me to do so.

I made my first therapy appointment with an enormous sense of guilt—but also with profound feelings of relief—and walked into that session with tears streaming uncontrollably down my cheeks. At last, I could admit to feeling utterly *lost.*

I did not tell my parents about this new development until six months later. I knew they would feel threatened by the idea of my discussing my famous father with someone in his own profession, and I was anxious about presenting them with the fait accompli. But one weekend when we were visiting with them at their summer house on Cape Cod, I told them that I had been seeing a therapist for some months and that I was finding it enormously helpful. They were startled and alarmed, as I had known they would be, but they accepted my reassurances that I had found a capable therapist whom I trusted to maintain confidentiality about the family issues I was revealing to him. To my parents' great credit, they quickly saw the importance of my having made this decision for myself, and respected my reasons. Very likely they sensed a change in me as well—the very beginnings of a new self-assurance—and that would have been gratifying to them, indeed. Their response was as generous and supportive as my parents always wanted to be.

Ironically, it was in the process of seeking help that I eventually began to appreciate one of the most precious gifts my parents had given me: I had been blessed not only with a deep faith in the value of psychoanalytic insight, but also with a basic trust in the psychoanalytic process—a trust inspired, first of all, by an identification with my father. But ultimately, it was the loving effort on the part of both Mom and Dad to be better parents than their own that had made it possible for me to benefit profoundly from a source of healing to which neither of them had been able to turn—even in their darkest hours.

Chapter 7

New Beginnings

Starting Therapy

Being an analytic patient was the first occupation I had ever fully embraced. I knew at once that this was where the answers lay for me, though I had no idea what they were. When people asked me during the next few years, "What do you do?" I was tempted to answer, "I'm in therapy." It was the only thing, besides motherhood, to which I felt fully committed.

But even in my acute state of need, it was not easy getting started. I felt, inevitably, that I was betraying my parents, who had sacrificed so much for so long to maintain secrecy about the sources of their shame. The importance of secrecy and of maintaining a public image had been so paramount in my family life that talking openly (and to someone in my father's own profession!) about my experience of my parents felt deeply disloyal. Unconsciously, and to some extent consciously as well, I feared that I had the power to destroy them and that my revelations about them to an outsider were a callous form of murder. I'm sure this fear lay behind many lapses in memory on my part—aspects of the family story that I "forgot" to talk about in the early months of treatment. Ultimately, it may have been a relief *and* a disappointment to discover that my words were not nearly as powerful as I had imagined.

But more important, if I had always felt like a peripheral figure in my parents life rather than the central figure in my own life, how was I ever to feel like the central character in my own therapy? Was I, in my own right, of any genuine importance to my therapist? Or was I primarily a source of information about my father, who was an icon in my therapist's own profession? In one of the few dreams I remember from that long-ago time:

> I arrive at a party where a man, whom I know, greets me and tells me he would like to meet my father. It seems that my father is already there, but the two of them haven't yet been introduced. I take this man to meet my father, and the two of them become deeply absorbed in conversation. Neither shows any further interest in me and I wander away.

DOI: 10.4324/9781003645757-8

I sobbed as I reported this dream to my therapist, so convinced that my worst fears about his essential disinterest in *me* were about to be confirmed. And I remember the profound sense of relief that swept over me when I was somehow assured that my fear, though entirely natural, was based on a distorted view of reality. My therapist acknowledged his own curiosity about my father and his emotional reaction to hearing about the human underside of fame, but he also convinced me of his genuine concern for the way the family drama had affected *me* and for the pain I was now expressing. Though we had already been meeting for many weeks by this time, my therapist acknowledged the special importance of my dream and of this session by remarking as I left his office that he thought we were "well begun."

There were other dreams that opened up pervasive themes in my emotional life. I have mentioned before the dream in which I had Mongolian features (resembled a person from Mongolia) and had to recognize my long-standing identification with Neil, who had been labeled, in the terminology of the 1940s, a Mongolian idiot.

I also had countless dreams about the inadequacy of the food I was able to provide to others or to myself, and the relative superiority of other women's food (all of them symbolizing, of course, my incomparable mother). Such dreams reflected anxiety about my essential ability to nurture—an ability that had been brought painfully into question when I became a mother. I was finding it agonizingly difficult to tolerate the dependency needs of my small son—agonizing because I wanted so desperately to be a good mother to him and yet resented the claims he made on me at a time when I was so conflicted about my own dependency needs. I imagined that my intolerance made me irrevocably different from, and inferior to, my own mother—the paragon (in my eyes) of maternal caregiving. It was several years before I began to recognize, ever so slowly, how much my struggles as a mother reflected the ways in which I had felt deeply deprived as a child—because of my mother's difficulty tolerating *my* dependency on *her.* I had to begin to acknowledge without shame my own thwarted needs before I could be more the kind of mother I desperately wanted to be. And it was only then that the dreams about the inadequacy of my "food" abated.

But the most prevalent dream theme during the first decade of my therapy/analysis related to the terrifying process of climbing down from some very high and precarious place (a mountain, a ladder, a cliff, a monument, a muddy slope, an "ivory tower," a pedestal, a statue, a roof, or a tall tree) to get my feet firmly on the ground. These dreams always evoked feelings of terror. Clearly, the high ground to which my parents had retreated for their own emotional safety—the realm of grandiosity, idealization, and fame—felt lonely and terribly *unsafe* to me. But that did not mean it was easy to come down from that lofty place—to let go of my own narcissistic defenses (the thought that I was secretly as special as my parents). Coming down to earth promised me much greater safety in the long run: I would feel less compelled to hide my feelings of shame and self-doubt and could, by acknowledging and expressing them, gain genuine relief at last. But getting my feet on the ground also exposed my human flaws and emotional vulnerability in a way my parents had never been able to tolerate—in themselves or in me.

This was the conflict that pervaded my dream life for many years as I searched for the solid ground between a grandiose sense of self (the Erikson in me) and feelings of utter worthlessness (also an inheritance, paradoxically, from my illustrious parents). The struggle to accept myself on a human level—flaws, vulnerabilities, and all—still gives me nightmares from time to time, and I'm sure it always will. But the more this struggle has become part of my conscious awareness, the less it has needed expression in my dreams.

On the other side of that struggle was the fear that by owning my own abilities and strengths, I would "disempower" my parents. As odd as that may sound coming from the daughter of my mother and father, I have since learned how pervasive this fear is in all of us, representing one of the most powerful obstacles to emotional growth and development. When we discover in ourselves strengths and abilities that seem to threaten our parents' hegemony over us, it often feels as if we have dethroned them—a frightening prospect, indeed. We are never ready to get along entirely without the internalized image of our parents as more powerful than ourselves and therefore able to make the world safe for us.

In a dream that occurred well into my analysis

> I look through a doorway into a room that has a large picture window. Outside the window is a fantastic view of a meadow and snow-capped mountain, with sunlight gleaming on the snow. I wonder whether this view could possibly be real, since I have not seen it from my own room in the same house. Maybe it is just a mural or some other kind of fake image. I rush over to the window to see for myself whether the scene is real. A woman sitting at a desk in the room reprimands me for disturbing an electrical cord which goes from the wall socket to her desk. She says the flow of electricity to her desk was disturbed as I went by. I don't believe I really touched the cord, but I become cautious and step over it carefully. When I look out the window again, the mountain scene is gone and there is a small garden outside with high walls around it. As I leave the room, I say, "Oh, I remember that garden. I went to a party there during my adolescence."

I have never doubted that the woman in that dream is (perhaps among other figures) my mother, and that in my unconscious, a discovery of new vistas for myself has the potential to disrupt her source of power. This is just what *seems* to have happened in my early adolescence when I began to be attractive and popular, resulting in my exile from the family home. And it is one of the fears that inhibited my career ambition for several decades of my adult life.

Ultimately, my mother surprised me with her genuine enthusiasm when I finally *did* embark on a career as a psychoanalyst. She was in her mid-eighties at the time, and I'm not at all sure that she could have enjoyed my professional emanation much earlier in her life.

My Years of Living Dangerously

A year or so after my analytic exploration had begun, Harley and I separated. The process was wrenching for both of us and even worse, of course, for Per. But I was driven by the need for an entirely different kind of life from that Harley and I had shared (and from the kind of life my parents had shared). I renounced academia entirely, dropping out of graduate school with an inordinate sense of relief that I no longer needed to pretend to be an intellectual—convinced now that I was not one and never had been. I chose friends and dated men who had little or no connection with academia. I went dancing and spent weekends with the singles crowd on Fire Island (a lovely spit of land reachable only by boat from Long Island) or in the Catskills. It was the kind of heady adolescent experience I had enjoyed so briefly at The Stockbridge School before I was sent away to Putney, and now *nothing* was going to deprive me of the opportunity. New York City and environs offered just the sense of anonymity I needed to dispel my concern for the family image and allowed me to enjoy both the social and the sexual freedom that attended the postadolescent single life.

In addition, it was now possible to have friendships more intimate than any I had experienced in the past, since I was so much less fearful of revealing my own or my family's secrets. Conversations with my closest friends were more candid than any I had participated in earlier in my life, often centering on our efforts to understand ourselves and others more fully, and on books that we found helpful in this pursuit.

It was wonderful to be free of the agonizing perfectionism I had always brought to academic work—mine as well as Harley's. It was far less torturous to work as a secretary (1*administrative assistant* in the new terminology) to pay the rent and to share in the support of Per while I savored my social life—unconcerned whether the men I met were appropriate companions for the daughter of a famous psychoanalyst.

Paradoxically, I was also discovering that I had been programmed at an early age in the language of analysis and that it was the language I spoke best. All the years I had spent listening to conversations in the household of my childhood, all the ways in which my father thought about things and explained them to me, and even (though it is still difficult for me to admit it) all that I had learned from reading his books—these were the early influences that now came to the fore in my emotional and intellectual awakening, and that helped me to make sense of my experience, past and present. Altogether, it was a very exciting time.

The saddest part, of course, was the cost to Per of the separation and divorce. There was no denying the pain this inflicted on him, and my grief and sense of guilt about this was sometimes overwhelming to me. Harley and I both did our best to ease the transition for Per, making sure he spent ample time with his dad, though he continued to live with me. Harley had always doted on Per and continued, as he has to this day, to be an involved and adoring father.

And as my psychotherapy progressed, I began to derive enormous gratification from my relationship with Per—one of the greatest rewards for me of the analytic process.

Visiting in Cotuit

By the time Harley and I separated in the early 1970s, my parents had moved from Cambridge back to Stockbridge, Massachusetts (for a brief period), and then to Tiburon, California. During this time, they still maintained their summer house in Cotuit on Cape Cod, where Per and I visited them often. Kai and his wife, Jo, had built a house on a lot adjacent to our parents', so summer was also a time for family gatherings with them and their children, Keith and Christopher.

Dad was an affectionate but distant grandfather, unsure how to relate to his grandchildren, but Mother thrilled to her role. After all, it was her own grandmother who had made her feel uniquely cherished when she was a child. It gave her enormous pleasure to pass that gift on to her children's children.

I remember those years as the most enjoyable in my relationship to my parents. I no longer looked to them in the same way for clues as to how I should be, and I was becoming increasingly confident about the ways in which I did *not* want to be like them. Especially important, I realize in retrospect, was my growing awareness that Mother had not been such a perfect mother after all. This revelation enhanced my confidence in my own mothering abilities (which had already benefited very much from my analytic work) and also allowed me to appreciate her generosity to me as well as to Per as we coped with the aftermath of the divorce. In fact, I was becoming freer to appreciate the many qualities in both my parents and their lifestyle that I *did* admire and want to emulate.

At the same time, the obvious changes in my sense of well-being were very gratifying to Mom and Dad. They had not known how to help me find my way, but they were thrilled that I had embarked on this process for myself.

Dad Comes Under Fire

I was so focused on the challenges of my new life in New York that I was not fully aware of the ways in which Dad's reputation was being seriously challenged in the mid-1970s. He had been widely revered since the publication of *Childhood and Society* in 1950, but public acclaim always brings with it negative as well as positive recognition. And as Dad's fame grew, he became the target of more and more intense criticism. Right from the beginning, it was inevitable, for example, that his mentors in Vienna would consider his work to be a betrayal of the Freudian theory to which they had introduced him. Unlike Freud, Dad emphasized the importance of cultural influences in human psychological development, and he was outspoken in his criticism of Freudians for giving so little importance to sociocultural factors. He hoped, of course, that this expansion in perspective might be appreciated by those who had introduced him to psychoanalysis—most importantly, his own analyst, Anna Freud. The few times that Dad had anticipated seeing Ms. Freud again years after he had left his analysis with her in Vienna, he was exceptionally anxious and hopeful of some theoretical reconciliation. But though she was polite and diplomatic in her face-to-face encounters with him, she never indicated real acceptance of his ideas. She considered him a renegade whose work was therefore not of great value—a particularly painful rejection for him.

At the same time, others thought that Dad's work did not *break clearly enough* with Freudian theory, limiting its contribution to contemporary psychoanalytic thought. Though he was, and continues to be, credited with a uniquely important psychoanalytic perspective, he did not make the sort of radical break from Freud that put some of his contemporaries on the psychoanalytic map (Donald W. Winnicott, W.R.D. Fairbairn, Harry Stack Sullivan, and Heinz Kohut, to name a few). And so, despite his success in reaching a much wider public than most of his contemporaries, and despite his status as something of an intellectual hero in the wider culture, Dad felt marginalized in relation to the new schools of thought gaining predominance in modern psychoanalysis (for example, object relations theory, interpersonal theory, and self psychology).

In addition, Dad's work had come under vigorous attack from feminists during the 1960s because of an article he wrote concerning differences in the play constructions of little boys and little girls. His focus on gender differences in this piece was interpreted as condoning and legitimating social inequality between the sexes. The breadth of the criticism grew as Dad was called to task for the gender bias inherent in his theory of the eight stages of the life cycle. It was argued that his developmental theory described the life cycle of men more accurately than the life cycle of women, emphasizing the masculine values of separation and independence to the neglect of the more relational orientation of women. Dad was always somewhat bewildered by this critique, believing that he was himself a feminist, and that he had been misunderstood and erroneously stereotyped.

What wounded my father most deeply of all was an attack on his authenticity as a man and as a theorist that appeared in the *New York Times Book Review* in 1975. A Jewish intellectual by the name of Marshall Berman, a professor of political science at City College of New York and a former Harvard graduate student who had attended Dad's graduate seminar during the 1960s, wrote a scathing review of Dad's book *Life History and the Historical Moment.* Most striking, he accused Dad of concealing his Judaism both by changing his surname from Homburger to Erikson and by failing to reveal publicly that his mother was Jewish. Berman accused Dad of a personal lack of authenticity, suggesting that this personal weakness brought into question the very concept of identity—the conceptual core, in some ways, of Dad's contribution to contemporary thought. The review ended by asserting that Dad's own self-image was "built on systematic repression and 'noble' lies."

It is ironic that this attack came from a direction Dad never expected. Yet it penetrated deeply. It exposed his life-long uncertainty about his parentage—the shame associated with having been abandoned by his father and not knowing who his father was. It exposed Dad's desire to dissociate himself from his Jewish stepfather, and it also exposed the extent to which his own identity was rooted in the fantasy that his biological father was a Danish Gentile, though the truth of this had never been firmly established. Ultimately, of course, the identity of Dad's biological father had no technical bearing on Dad's ethnicity, which was determined, according to Jewish law, by the fact that his mother was Jewish.

To be accused of fraudulence is always acutely painful, but this attack was particularly devastating in its exposure of unresolved identity issues in a man famous for bringing the concepts of identity and identity crisis, to the fore not only in psychoanalytic thought but also in the culture as a whole. In his biography of Dad, Lawrence Friedman acknowledges that "several of Erikson's closest friends and family realized that [Berman] was not wholly off the mark" in his identification of Dad's deepest uncertainties about himself.

What made this critique more difficult to accept was that Dad was discouraged by his longtime editor, George Brockway, from writing a letter in his own defense to the editor of the *Book Review.* Other friends and advisers (including Kai) agreed that it was best for Dad not to respond directly to Berman, leaving Dad to feel painfully revealed on the public stage.

I remember this as a difficult time for my parents, but I underestimated the seriousness of the matter, partly because my own life was by then so far removed from the intellectual world, and partly because they did not admit in my presence to being as devastated by these attacks as they really were. But I do remember that Dad spent a good deal of time writing (and compulsively rewriting) letters and memoranda to relatives and friends, trying desperately to explain himself. One letter to his half-sister Ruth, dated April 16, 1975, reads

> I hope you know that when I changed my name at the time of my naturalization procedure (as millions have done), both Muts [their mother] and Papa [Ruth's father and his stepfather] agreed. I then did not expect someday to have "a name" with all its consequences, good and bad.
>
> Well, try to forgive me.

Mother responded to this crisis with a characteristic dismissal of Berman and the review as preposterously unfair and unworthy of rebuttal. She did her best to reassure Dad that this critique was unimportant in the larger scheme of things and would not be taken seriously by anyone who admired his work. But she was not entirely correct about this. Dad's public reputation *was* damaged. Friedman reports that sales of his books plummeted in the year after the essay was published, and never again achieved their previous heights.

It is quite likely, of course, that Dad's book sales had run their course and that the decline in sales immediately following Berman's review reflected not only a reaction to this critique but also a natural and inevitable diminution of interest in Dad's work after his twenty-five years of exceptional prominence. But Dad never quite recovered from this assault on his personal, as well as his intellectual, integrity.

At the same time, he was now more marginalized professionally as a consultant, first at Riggs in Stockbridge and later at Mt. Zion Hospital in San Francisco, having retired from full-time work. He never seemed as satisfied again with his level of involvement in institutional settings, and clearly missed the special status he had enjoyed both at Riggs in the 1950s and at Harvard in the 1960s.

The 1980s

I had been separated for six years by the time I met Bob in 1980 at a singles resort in the Catskills. This is not where I had expected to meet Mr. Right, but almost nothing about my life in the previous decade had been what I had expected, so nothing was now beyond my wildest imagination. Before meeting Bob, I had made no conscious decision to bring my single life to an end, and it was not a transition I was eager to make. But this relationship demanded serious consideration, and that is what compelled me to turn the next corner in my life.

Bob was a lawyer (now retired) and won Per's heart the first time they met by taking him to play video games. It was clear within a short period of time that all three of us thrived on this new connection with each other, and so the decision seemed to make itself. Bob moved in with Per and me in 1981. His two daughters, Jessica and Jillian (who lived with their mother in New Jersey), spent many weekends with us in our New York City apartment during the next eight years, and we often traveled together to see relatives in different parts of the country (Bob's mother in Kansas City and my parents in Cotuit or in Tiburon, California). Both Per and I reveled in this taste of family life.

During this period, neither Bob nor I felt deeply invested in our work. Our relationship was more important to both of us than the hours we spent earning a living—a radical change for me, and a deeply gratifying one, from the lifestyle of my parents.

But when all three of our kids had left for college, I was suddenly overwhelmed with dissatisfaction at my lack of interest in my work life. It was a shock to discover that my employment as a secretary, which had seemed to serve me well while I was actively engaged as a mother, no longer made sense to me after Per and the girls had left home. I felt without purpose, and I knew it was time to find a more gratifying way to spend my days *and* make a living.

On a beautiful September day, just two weeks after Per had started college, I decided to walk to my therapy session—a distance of more than eighty city blocks. Brisk walking always makes me feel more courageous than I feel when I am sedentary, and somewhere in the course of that marathon, three undeniable realities came together in my thoughts: I had a pressing need for more intellectual stimulation; I wanted to earn more money; *and* I had a natural ease with, and love for, psychoanalytic exploration. It was time to think about becoming a psychotherapist. The therapy session that followed that brisk walk was all that was needed to seal my fate.

And so it was that, filled with trepidation, I entered the enchanted land where my father was king—if not a god—and where I knew I would have to face the most terrifying of my own monsters: the humiliation of being a commoner in my father's glorious kingdom, and (paradoxically) the fear of triggering in myself the kind of addictive ambition that would damage my most cherished relationships. It is not surprising that my years of clinical training were emotionally tumultuous at the same time that they were deeply gratifying.

The continued analysis required as part of my training helped me very gradually to find my own psychoanalytic identity. But I also chose this critical moment to join a psychotherapy group, which was to play a key part over the next fifteen years in helping me to struggle with the issues posed by my decision to become an analyst. In the context of this therapy group, I confronted, over and over again, the stultifying effect of my father's fame on my sense of myself and of my own capabilities as I strived to feel worthy of my own career in psychoanalysis. I found that revealing myself as openly as possible to a group of people who identified with many of my feelings, or were at least empathic with them even when my personal demons were different from theirs, helped enormously to reduce my feelings of inadequacy and to make me feel more acceptable to others in my own right—personal flaws, vulnerabilities, and all.

Where my parents felt compelled to hide the shame of their early trauma behind a public image of confidence and near perfection, I was given the opportunity to acknowledge and to *reveal* my worst feelings about myself—to expose them to the light of day time after time, session after session—and to experience the relief that such exposure can provide. This offered a powerful alternative to the suffering I had witnessed in my parents' lives, and which I had shared with them as a child. But I understand now why this form of relief was more available to me than it had been to my parents. I had had a far more nurturing childhood than had either of them, and I was better able to trust both the analytic process and the people who sought to help me.

It was in this therapeutic setting as well that I struggled with my fear of ambition: the belief that it might consume me (as it had my parents) if I became more confident of my ability and allowed myself to seek professional recognition at all. In the context of group therapy, I gradually came to trust that I would never allow ambition to deprive me of the intimacy I had longed for as a child and young adult. At the same time, the group's supportive acceptance of my professional successes provided the reassurance I needed that accomplishment, in and of itself, would not isolate me from those with whom I shared genuine intimate connection. I believe that this profound therapeutic experience, more than any other, clarified for me the difference between my parents' way of being in the world and what I wanted most for myself.

It does not escape me, of course, that what my parents *did* with their unhealed childhood wounds was of immeasurable value to the world, whereas my own pursuit of a less anguished life promises no such contribution to human civilization. But I am deeply grateful, nevertheless, for the sources of healing that have been made available to me.

My years in analysis and group therapy have by no means cured me of the deepest conflicts engendered by my family experience, but they have made it possible for me to confront them more directly, as I did in embarking on a career in my father's field. And they helped me to discover a connection with my father that would have been much too frightening for me to acknowledge without the benefit of prior self-exploration: an appreciation for his way of understanding the human psyche and his humane perspective on the human condition. What I had internalized of Dad's analytic perspective was to become an invaluable asset to me as an analyst, and eventually helped me to better understand *him,* and my mother as well—the two biggest mysteries in the universe of my personal experience.

Chapter 8

Becoming a Psychoanalyst

I began my training in the late 1980s. Knowing at the outset that my goal was to become a clinician, I chose the shortest and most direct path to obtaining a respected credential in the field: a master's degree in social work. The alternative—a Ph.D. in psychology—would have taken years longer and would have prepared me for activities in which I did not plan to engage—most importantly, scholarly research, teaching, and writing. A master's in social work, by contrast, can be completed in two years and combines academic work with direct clinical experience (obtained through internships in social work/mental health agencies) for both of those years.

As a social work student at New York University (whose program offers training specifically in clinical social work), I interned first in a mental health clinic that offered outpatient treatment for the chronically mentally ill and, second, in an inpatient unit of a mental hospital where the patients were in an acute state of crisis.

From the first day of my training in this field, it was as though everything I had done during the years of my career avoidance had prepared me for this enterprise. Not only had I been introduced to an analytic perspective early in my life, but I had also spent nearly fifteen years in therapy by this time, and this personal exploration had opened up worlds of understanding not only of myself, but of others as well. I had also spent countless hours in the classroom studying anthropology and sociology, and had written innumerable term papers. Classroom work was only too familiar to me. The surprise was that clinical work felt uncannily familiar too. But here I confronted—all at the same time—my greatest strengths and my deepest insecurities.

There was, first of all, the perfectionism that had haunted all my earlier efforts in the academic realm. Although I had both the psychological *and* the sociological background to do well in social work courses, I worked too hard on each and every term paper, even knowing (at least intellectually) that a perfect academic record was of minimal importance in my pursuit of a clinical career. What drove this perfectionism was the lurking humiliation of being found wanting in even the smallest way—a disgrace, in the Erikson family tradition, to be avoided at all cost.

Naturally, this anxiety pervaded my performance in the social work internships as well. An evaluation I received from my second-year supervisor noted my "fear of not being perfect," but indicated that by the middle of that year, I finally seemed to be more confident of my real abilities and had begun to be less self-critical.

DOI: 10.4324/9781003645757-9

And, of course, there was my long-standing insecurity about being able to nourish—to take care of—others. This self-doubt had been greatly diminished in the course of my own therapy, but such deep personal issues don't ever go entirely away. Under new circumstances and pressures, they can always resurface. And this one did, expressing itself in a dream the night after I met with my first clinic patient. The dream consisted of just one image: a millipede-like insect that had attached itself to my leg, with all its legs dug into my flesh. This image conveyed the unconscious terror I still felt at allowing people to become dependent on me—at inviting them to need something from me that I was not sure I could provide.

Finally, there was my reluctance to exercise authority. My mother was, after all, the unquestioned authority in the home of my childhood, and my ambivalence toward her dictatorial ways had complicated my relationship with my own assertiveness. On the one hand, I had not dared to challenge her judgment about what was best for all of us. To assert my own will, as a child, was to disrupt the precarious bond between Mother and me and risk losing the caretaking I longed for from her and thought of as indispensable to my well-being. On the other side of the coin, however, was my resentment of Mother's controlling ways, and the fear that in wielding any authority myself I would become just like her—potentially just as controlling as she was. This anxiety had played an important part in my early decision to become a secretary, a role where I would take orders and almost never have to give them.

But both of my social work internships required that I assume a leadership role in relation to clients. In the first instance, I was called upon to co-lead, and occasionally lead, groups of chronically mentally ill patients, an assignment requiring that I establish firm boundaries and remain—however benevolently—in control. In my second year, I met with the families of patients just admitted to a mental hospital for the acutely mentally ill—families who were typically distraught, bewildered, and/or angry at being told that one of their members (a parent, a child, or a sibling) was, in fact, very ill and in need of psychiatric care. Again, the challenge was to remain firmly in control while helping people to cope with the difficult realities of mental illness. In both these instances, my ability to do the job was clear to my supervisors and the rest of the professional staff before it was clear to me. But by the end of these internships, I felt much more capable of exercising authority without becoming the compulsively controlling or domineering woman I had always feared in myself.

I also faced another challenge to my sense of self during the second year: presenting family case histories to the psychiatric staff of the hospital at rounds. The first time I was asked to prepare such a case for presentation, I experienced again the momentary feeling that there must be some mistake. This was not the sort of professional authority I had ever before exercised. Once again, my supervisor and other members of the staff saw the appropriateness of the assignment well before it became apparent to me. And it was in fulfilling their expectations that I discovered in myself a natural ability that surprised no one but me.

Twenty years earlier, in his biography of my father *(Erik H. Erikson: The Growth of His Work),* Robert Coles had described me as "a very bright and able scholar, yet in mind as well as manner ... very much a certain kind of woman: quietly wise and intellectually giving rather than argumentative and self-assertive." When I graduated from the M.S.W. program at NYU, I felt like a very different kind of woman from the one so described.

But such momentous transitions are never made without psychological repercussions, and—not surprisingly as I look back on it—I was depressed for several months after this combination of internships had ended. I had invaded my father's territory and had felt well respected there for my own abilities. I had challenged my mother's authority with my new assertiveness. Psychologically speaking, I had become a bit bigger in the universe, whereas my parents had become a bit smaller; and I mourned the loss of the seemingly omnipotent caretakers of my childhood.

In fact, these internships were not the only context in which my internal map of the world was being revised. I was also beginning to learn, for the first time, about the history of psychoanalytic theory and my father's place in it. Through all my years of self-exploration in psychotherapy, and despite all the books I had read about the workings of the human psyche, I had never been terribly interested in the theoretical controversies that had dominated the history of psychoanalysis. So one semester at NYU, I did an independent study project in which I explored for the first time the relationship between Freudian theory and the schools of psychoanalytic thought that have come more recently to the fore. As belated as this inquiry was for me, it gave me a basic sense of the psychoanalytic map and of my father's place on that map.

I learned that Dad's work continued to be important in two areas in particular. His model of the eight stages of human development was still considered useful in child psychoanalysis as well as in the field of developmental psychology, where it had focused new attention on the importance of adult development. Dad was the first, in fact, to propose that adulthood could be conceptualized in terms of stages of development, just as childhood had been by earlier theorists, including Freud. Implicit in the earlier focus on childhood was the assumption that little significant personality change occurs after the formative years, so adulthood needed little theoretical attention. Dad's model emphasized what is now taken widely for granted: the potential for significant change and growth throughout the life cycle.

And just as important, Dad's books on Martin Luther *(Young Man Luther)* and Gandhi *(Gandhi's Truth)* had stimulated critical new developments in the field of psychohistory, which focuses on the relationship between individual psychology and sociocultural environment in the study of innovative figures in world history.

For all of Dad's continued importance in these areas of psychoanalysis, he was not considered to be the founder of a new school of thought. By contrast, some of his contemporaries, whose writing style is less accessible and less widely captivating than his—and who are, therefore, less well known outside the field—*are* considered to be the founders of new movements in American psychoanalysis: for example, Harry Stack Sullivan (the father of interpersonal theory) and Heinz Kohut (the father of self psychology). Although they are less "famous" than my father, both of these innovators have, nonetheless, had a more profound impact on the way in which the human psyche is conceptualized in contemporary theory, and the way in which psychoanalysis is practiced.

It was Freud's view that the most basic elements of the human psyche—the drives (sex, aggression, the pursuit of pleasure, for instance)—are inborn and essentially biological in nature. Similarly, he believed that the structure of the psyche—its organization into an id, an ego, and a superego—was inborn rather than a product of interpersonal experience. In Freudian theory, the family environment plays a part in directing or inhibiting the way the drives are expressed—and therefore in determining how the psyche will develop—but what is innate in the psyche plays an equal (if not greater) role in determining personality.

Dad's work departed from Freud in his greater emphasis on the importance of the interpersonal environment in shaping personality, and he was considered particularly innovative for his insights concerning the impact of the larger social and cultural milieu on psychological development. But he did not completely abandon Freud's drive-based theory of development or Freud's concept of the psyche as having an innate structure. (Dad's model of the life cycle delineated psychosocial stages in contrast to Freud's psychosexual stages of development, but this schema paralleled Freud's model rather than replaced it.)

By contrast, Harry Stack Sullivan (among other subsequent theorists), rejected Freud's drive theory outright, emphasizing the impact of interpersonal relationships not only on the way personality develops, but also on the very origin of the psyche and the nature of its most basic contents. Rather than assuming the existence of drives and a structure of mind that predate any experience of the interpersonal world, Sullivan suggested that the personality is entirely a product of interpersonal experience, beginning with the infant's first interactions with his or her caretakers. Today, this assumption is fundamental not only to interpersonal theory but to other contemporary schools of thought as well. It underlies a significant segment of what has been characterized as the "relational" perspective in psychoanalysis.

A concomitant of the relational perspective is a new way of thinking about the psychoanalytic process. If the psyche is in important measure the product of interpersonal relationships, then the most important source of change in the functioning of the personality is through engagement in a new kind of relationship—namely, the relationship between patient and psychoanalyst. Freud had prescribed that the analyst remain neutral in his posture toward the patient—a "blank slate" whose personality is revealed as little as possible. From this neutral position, the analyst could then interpret the material brought to him by the patient, producing change by making clear to the patient why he felt the way he felt or did what he did. Interpretation—or insight—was considered the curative factor in the interaction between patient and analyst. (It has often been pointed out that although this was what Freud *said* about the nature of analysis, it is not what he himself *did*. By his own description of his relationships with patients, he was far from a blank slate.

From the relational perspective, however, the relationship between the analyst and patient is a key curative factor. Interpretation and insight, while indispensable, are thought to derive their power from the relationship within which they arise. Furthermore, it is argued it is impossible for anyone to be a blank slate in the context of the analytic relationship, no matter how hard the analyst might try. Human beings reveal themselves unconsciously as well as consciously in every interaction with others. An analyst who believes that he has not revealed himself to the patient is simply denying the reality of his constant self-exposure. So the only authentic stance for an analyst to take is to admit at the outset to being fundamentally human—albeit specially trained for the work at hand—and to make his or her subjective experience of the analytic relationship part of the process to be examined. Reading about this trend in modern psychoanalysis, I realized for the first time that the analysts with whom I had been in treatment had *all* embraced the interpersonal perspective. All of them had been more actively engaged, more emotionally present, and self-revealing in their work with me, than I would ever have expected given my family background. My experience of these analytic relationships had been deeply gratifying and life enhancing in contrast to the way in which both my parents had kept themselves emotionally hidden. And once I understood the theoretical underpinnings of my analytic experience, it was only too clear that I wanted to be trained as an interpersonal analyst myself—that I would not be gratified by any other kind of relationship with my own patients. The next step after the M.S.W. degree would be training at an interpersonal psychoanalytic institute.

Dad's Decline

By the time I began working toward my M.S.W. in the late 1980s, my parents were again living in Cambridge, Massachusetts. Immediately following my father's heyday at Harvard in the 1960s, they had returned briefly to Stockbridge, and then settled on the West Coast—in Tiburon, California—fully expecting to retire there. What was not expected was that my father would begin to withdraw—emotionally and cognitively—sometime in the middle of the 1980s, first finding it difficult to write, and then difficult to read other people's writing as well. His ability to converse became more limited as his memory slowly failed. I never heard a formal diagnosis applied to his gradual decline (which did not resemble Alzheimer's), but it seemed as though he had finally succumbed to the depression that had haunted his life.

In the late 1980s, my parents were invited by two younger colleagues to share a house with them in Cambridge, close to the Harvard campus, where Mom would have their help in caring for Dad. This arrangement promised not only to lighten the burden of caretaking for Mom but also to provide her with the intellectual companionship that was now missing in her relationship with Dad. And so my parents moved back to Cambridge in 1988.

As I made my own entry into the world of psychoanalysis, Dad had already withdrawn almost entirely from the intellectual realm. I am not at all sure that I could have embarked on the journey while my father was still actively engaged in his career. And for more reasons than one. Most obviously, his prominence in the field would have been overwhelming to me had he continued to attract wide public attention while I was just trying my wings. But just as important, though less obvious, I would have found it difficult to share with him the extent to which I was not going to be following in his theoretical footsteps.

In my youth, when I had resisted reading Dad's books, I had known that he was eager for me to do so. It was Mother who had made me particularly aware of this, suggesting that I read the books for his sake as well as for my own. And Dad, in acknowledging that he had been an inattentive father, expressed the hope that I would nevertheless be nourished by what he had written. So my eventual allegiance to other schools of analytic thought more than to my father's work caused me considerable anxiety—even after he was no longer able to comprehend the betrayal. Several years into my training, I dreamed that

> I have had two meetings with a man who seems to want me to read something—an article or some notes he has written. I have been analyzing his request but not taking the material from him. He tells me in the presence of other people how much pain I have caused him by not reading the notes as he had asked me to. He puts his face very close to mine and it is contorted with pain and rage. I have failed him catastrophically. I say, "I didn't mean to cause you such pain!" and it comes from deep in my gut.

For all my feelings of guilt about not embracing Dad's work, the truth is that I have always been more interested in trying to understand *him as a person* than in trying to understand what he wrote. Notice that in the dream, I am "analyzing his request" rather than taking the written material from him. I have wanted to understand my father's drive to write, his need for me (and the rest of the world) to read his work—his need for fame—as a way of coming to terms with the distance created between us by his preoccupation with achievement. This desire to understand him became a guiding force in my eventual focus, as an analyst, on issues relating to the pursuit of fame.

I was able to tell Dad, after the decision was first made in the late 1980s, that I was going to become a psychoanalyst. It was still possible, at that time, to have limited conversation with him, and his response was deeply touching: "That's wonderful!" he said, with a sweet and joyful smile. I like to think that he grasped the real meaning of this decision: that for all my resistance to reading his books, I *did* cherish his way of understanding the world around him, and I was ready to embrace his way of looking at things.

Psychoanalytic Training

A master's degree in social work does not, in itself, prepare a person to engage in clinical work. There is, first of all, a state examination to be passed following the completion of the degree, and it is this exam that leads to state certification (in effect, a license) as a clinical social worker. Secondly, it is widely agreed in the field that such certification is only a stepping stone to further training as a clinician, which can be acquired in a variety of ways. One can be further trained, for example, in psychodynamic psychotherapy, in cognitive or behavioral therapy, or in family or group therapy; but probably the most extensive form of additional clinical training is psychoanalytic.

Certification as a psychoanalyst usually requires five years of training in a psychoanalytic institute, many of which are clustered in big cities on the East and West coasts and in Chicago. Such training not only develops one's clinical skills in general, but it also instills an analytic perspective different from that which guides the practice of psychotherapy. Both approaches seek to clarify psychodynamic patterns and issues that underlie the behavior of the patient. But psychoanalysis, more than psychotherapy, devotes persistent attention to the early experiences of the patient as a means of understanding his or her way of relating to people and circumstances in the present. And even more important, psychoanalysis focuses more than does any other clinical approach on the patient's way of relating *to the analyst.* The patient's perception of, and reaction to, the analyst is seen as a reflection of the kinds of relationships that have prevailed (and have been internalized) in his or her early family life. It is assumed, in fact, that all the most pervasive patterns that are played out in the patient's relationships outside the analytic setting will eventually emerge in the analytic relationship as well. Thus, the exploration of what happens in the analytic encounter becomes a unique source of insight not only into the patient's past, but also into his or her characteristic ways of relating to others in the present.

Furthermore—in interpersonal psychoanalysis particularly—developments in the relationship between patient and analyst are understood as a two-way street. The analyst's reactions to the patient are not assumed to be neutral or objective but are understood, rather, to be a reflection of the analyst's own personality—his *own* early experiences, his unconscious, and his adult patterns of relating. Consequently, the analysis of interactions between analyst and patient requires attention to the psychology of *both* participants. What distinguishes the analyst's role in this process is a hard-earned self-awareness (acquired through his or her own extensive analysis) as well as expertise in understanding the psychology of the patient.

Particularly because of the characteristic focus on the analytic relationship in the practice of psychoanalysis, several years (if not more) of personal analysis are required of all psychoanalytic candidates.

What's in a Name?

By the time I began psychoanalytic training, I had been engaged in the field for three years, and I was still not using my maiden name (as I do today) as a middle name. I had told everyone closely involved in my training who my father was, and I had shared that information with a few classmates whom I had come to know especially well in the M.S.W. program. But many of my instructors, and most of my fellow students, did not know of this connection. And it was still quite traumatic for me to mention it. I had entered a world in which my father's work was *very* well known, and reactions to his name were often dramatic. Whenever mention of my relationship to him caused too much excitement, it disrupted the normal flow of social interaction and left me feeling disconnected. Such excitement, as I have said earlier, has always threatened to make me a mere conduit of my father's magic—a role in which I disappear from sight.

But training at the Manhattan Institute for Psychoanalysis involved five years of course work with a small class of candidates who progressed through the program together. Anonymity was out of the question. And having learned early on of my difficulty with this issue, my classmates urged me, with each new trimester, to reveal to our instructors my family background. The reaction in this context was consistently thoughtful and never felt disruptive or depersonalizing to me. It was as a member of this intimate and supportive class, and of the broader community of the institute, that I first began to feel comfortable with being identified as my father's daughter, and reclaimed the name Erikson as an integral part of my professional identity.

A Real Career

Psychoanalytic training requires a few hours of course work each week as well as clinical work with training cases, supervision, and one's own analysis. During the years of my training, I worked part time in a mental health clinic and developed my private practice. For the first time in my life, I gave myself over to a demanding schedule of work, and had no doubts about whether it was what I really wanted. After evening classes, I was frequently too stimulated to go to sleep. I was learning not only about the fascinating world of psychoanalytic ideas, but also about my instinctive connection with that world. And I had begun to make new and (to me) compelling connections between the ideas to which I was being introduced and the psychological phenomenon that had played such an important part in my life—namely, my father's fame.

I don't remember a particular moment when it occurred to me to focus my professional attention on issues relating to fame. But there were, indeed, critical moments in the course of my training when new insights and new opportunities combined to propel me in this direction. One such moment occurred during my very first year of study when I was asked to write a paper on a well-known personality of my choice. I had been fascinated by a television interview I had seen of Laurence Olivier a number of years earlier, and I decided to read his autobiography, *Confessions of an Actor*. This extraordinarily candid memoir stimulated not only a term paper about Olivier, but also a whole new way of thinking about my parents and their relationship to fame—in fact, a new way of thinking about the very nature of celebrity.

Chapter 9

Laurence Olivier

My fascination with Laurence Olivier actually goes back to 1983, when I saw a television interview he did with Barbara Walters. Walters asked him to explain a statement she had heard him make on a previous occasion: that he didn't like himself at all, that he didn't think he was a very nice man. "Well," Olivier replied, "I agree with me. I don't think I am. I just don't like me. I don't like my own company very much." Walters seemed stunned by this reassertion, clearly unable to imagine that a man such as Olivier could possibly dislike himself—especially since, she stated with final authority, he "couldn't be a nicer person."

I was as startled as Walters by Olivier's self-deprecating remarks—but not because I found it difficult to believe him. On the contrary, I felt he had been profoundly truthful about deeply rooted feelings of self-disapproval that lay hidden behind his larger-than-life facade—behind his image as a man of extraordinary talent, self-assurance, and charisma. I felt he had given voice to painful feelings of self-dislike much like those that haunted my father.

For Olivier to speak of these feelings so openly was shocking to me primarily because I had long believed that my father was the exception to the generally accepted rule that the achievement of fame brings self-acceptance and contentment. I had thought it abnormal that my father continued to feel inadequate despite the acclaim that had been heaped upon him. So it was astounding to me to hear that a man as monumentally successful as Laurence Olivier was plagued by feelings so similar to my father's.

Also, I had imagined until that moment that Olivier, whose physical presence on a stage was so powerfully dynamic and commanding, *must* be an emotional opposite to my father. I had been comparing my private experience of my father to the public image of Olivier. So I was especially astonished to learn that a man of Olivier's obvious confidence *in the exercise of his unique gifts* suffered from the same negative feelings about himself *personally* as did my father.

I was also taken aback that he would *admit* it. His candor about his personal suffering heightened my awareness of the dilemma that had haunted my relationship with my father. While Dad did not attempt to conceal his self-doubts in the context of his intimate relationships, he did not openly acknowledge to himself—or others—the depth of his feelings of personal inadequacy. When he confessed to me

DOI: 10.4324/9781003645757-10

once (he was in his sixties at the time) that he had been insecure as a young man, it was instantly clear to me that he did not know how profoundly his self-doubts continued to affect him and his closest relationships—how careful one had to be in his presence to avoid causing him the pain of self-recrimination. (And, of course, it would have seemed monstrous to me, at that unguarded moment, to bring this matter to his attention.) And so it seemed that Olivier had spoken the unspeakable—had defied all the rules I had internalized about what could safely be acknowledged to oneself or to others and what could not.

I certainly understood why no one (including Barbara Walters) found it easy to believe that someone like Olivier could possibly feel personally unworthy, given the immensity of his accomplishments, the charismatic way in which he related to his public, and the golden aura of fame that surrounded him. It is difficult for the admirers of a great man to imagine that the confidence he displays with respect to his special gifts can coexist with deep feelings of personal inadequacy.

Olivier confirmed that, indeed, they could; that my father's continued struggle with issues of self-acceptance, despite his illustrious achievements, was by no means unique; that self-disapproval can, in fact, persist—virtually unaffected—through the attainment of the most celebrated success.

So when I was asked in 1989 to write a paper about a well-known personality, I knew immediately who my subject would be. I turned to Olivier's *Confessions of an Actor* and found there that Olivier had struggled all his life with profound questions about his masculinity—with a sense that he was shamefully weak. He confesses to a lifelong sense of humiliation about the imperfections of his face, imperfections that were identified by an acting teacher who had said, "You have weakness … *here,*" as she ran her little finger down Olivier's forehead from the hairline to the top of his nose. Olivier "felt immediately the wisdom of this pronouncement" and began to seek refuge in theatrical facial disguises, without which he was never completely comfortable on the stage. Once, for example, he insisted on using nose putty in a performance with John Gielgud of *Romeo and Juliet,* though Gielgud *and* the director both begged him not to.

It was, of course, a *characterological* weakness that Olivier believed his face revealed; and his embarrassment about this glaring defect in his face and person endured throughout his great career.

Olivier also describes the enormous sense of guilt that sometimes overwhelmed him—as when his second wife, Vivien Leigh, succumbed to manic depression during their marriage. Someone more noble than himself, Olivier laments, might have been able to "bury … selfish thinking" and devote his remaining years to her; "but as will have been gathered by now, selfishness is almost like a gift with me." It is not incidental that his autobiography is entitled *Confessions of an Actor.* It is offered as a chronicle of his misdeeds, which begins with "Bless me, Reader, for I have sinned. Since my last confession, which was more than fifty years ago, I have committed the following sins …"

At the same time, of course, Olivier possessed a profound belief in his ability to win the attention of an audience. As an actor, he writes, "I have always had that rod of steel in my makeup; flexible, but there. I have always very much believed in myself, as of course every actor must."

Curious about the psychological origins of this emotional dichotomy, I found in *Confessions of an Actor* some profound similarities between Olivier's early life experience and that of both my father and my mother. Olivier was not physically abandoned by his father (as was my father), but he did feel profoundly rejected by him (much as both my parents had felt rejected as children). Olivier's father is reported to have felt a "sense of slight disgust" on first viewing his infant son—a disgust that seemed to Olivier to last all his boyhood.

His father's undisguised contempt made Olivier particularly vulnerable to rejection by others in his childhood environment. He was painfully unpopular as a young boy in public school, where he was universally referred to as "that sidey little shit Olivier," and was teased as a "tart" and a "flirt" because of his seductive mannerisms and his "pretty" face.

My parents, too, felt ostracized as children (albeit for different reasons). And they, like Olivier, had devoted themselves, in their loneliness, to solitary pursuits—seeking nourishment from passionate interests in the absence of the companionship that was not available to them. Olivier devoted himself obsessively to inventing plays and acting them out on a makeshift stage in the nursery. My father, of course, devoted himself to reading during those lonely early years. And mother sought adventure by land and by sea—on her bicycle, in the first instance, and in a small dinghy, in the second.

Both my father and Olivier were nurtured by a special bond with their mothers. My father's special relationship with his mother invited and supported his interest in reading and philosophy. Olivier's mother seems to have demonstrated undisguised favoritism toward "her Baby" (the youngest of her three children) and relished his dramatic performances in the nursery. As long as his mother was at home, Olivier remembers, he never "played to an empty house." She also campaigned to get him accepted into a prestigious boy's choir, subjecting him to countless humiliating auditions until he passed muster and even became the "solo-boy." Her ambition for her youngest son, like my grandmother's ambition for my father, was anything but a casual desire. She was driven by the need for vicarious gratification, which both women sought through their children's success.

But when Olivier was just twelve, his mother, "my heaven, my hope, my entire world, my own worshiped Mummy" died, leaving him in the care of his distant father. My parents, too, suffered early parental loss. And all three emerged from their childhood experiences with a driving need for recognition and acclaim. Writing of his boyhood longing for popularity, Olivier confesses that "the wish for this treacherous glory … has been obsessive all my life." Along with this ferocious appetite, he had a penchant for grandiose fantasy regarding the stardom he craved. He says quite simply of his early ambition, "My will was granite. I was determined to be the greatest actor of all time."

Many would claim that Olivier achieved this lofty goal. But within the account of his extraordinary success as an actor is evidence that his spectacular career failed to provide him with the sense of accomplishment that he so desperately longed for—accomplishment sufficient to free him from his deepest feelings of unworthiness. He reports having experienced great happiness during periods in his life when he was working at a frenetic pace—a pace he seems to have required to ward off feelings of depression. But he was rarely able to feel happy doing anything *other* than work. It was only in the exercise of his magical talent that Olivier experienced even momentary freedom from feelings of self-loathing.

And even his ability to perform was threatened on occasion by overwhelming anxiety. In both *Confessions of an Actor* and his second biography, *Laurence Olivier on Acting,* he chronicles the persistent fear that haunted his theatrical career—at times an "agonizing dread" as he approached each performance—that he would forget his lines or would become dizzy and fall. Worst of all, he was seriously debilitated for five and a half years (as he approached the age of sixty) by a prolonged attack of stage fright that threatened to bring his theatrical career to an end. Olivier connects this crisis in confidence with his perpetual fear of punishment for the grandiose ambition that had fueled his career and distracted him, at the same time, from being the attentive husband and father he felt he should have been.

Olivier did eventually overcome his paralyzing stage fright and continued acting until health problems ended his career. He was grateful for this brief reprieve, but was soon to find retirement punishing in its own way. He lamented in old age that "it is not easy to be put out to grass, left to feed on memories and friendships. An actor must act." His retirement was plagued by illness, to which he was particularly vulnerable because of the depression and anxiety that overwhelmed him—as it always had—when he was not working.

Though his autobiographical style is characteristically flamboyant, Olivier's extraordinary candor about his harshest feelings toward himself clarified for me the desperate struggle I had witnessed in both my parents to defend themselves against similarly harsh feelings of self-condemnation. Their vulnerability to shame and guilt was clearly revealed in the pattern of avoidance and denial with which they handled the crisis of Neil's birth, but this vulnerability had lurked behind their larger-than-life facade long before Neil came on the scene.

My parents' way of defending against feelings of personal inadequacy was, in one sense, the opposite of Olivier's. While they characteristically avoided acknowledging or discussing the issues that evoked in them the harshest feelings of self-reproach, Olivier's characteristic mode of defense was to broadcast these issues and feelings to the world along with passionate declarations of self-loathing and remorse. The potential disapproval of his audience was thus transformed into admiration for his candor and sympathy with his self-inflicted suffering. But as opposite as these defensive styles might seem, Olivier's self-revelation and my parents' secretiveness actually served the same psychological purpose.

My encounter with Olivier left me to wonder whether the two seemingly contradictory self-states that I had experienced in my father, and had now discovered in Olivier, could not only coexist but might actually be two sides of the same psychological coin. And, if so, what might this suggest about the nature of fame more generally?

Chapter 10

The Quest for Understanding

During the ten years following my paper on Laurence Olivier, I began to notice patterns in the self-revelations of famous people other than my father or Olivier that convinced me that these two figures were by no means unique in the world of celebrity. I noticed, for example, how often childhood trauma preceded the achievement of fame in most fields of human endeavor. And this threw into question all that I was learning about the disorganizing and disabling effects of trauma in children's early emotional development. Clearly, trauma made it more difficult for many children to function well or to achieve at all. Yet, for some, childhood tragedy seemed to provide a powerful impetus toward extraordinary accomplishment.

I had always been aware that certain cultural idols like Marilyn Monroe, Judy Garland, and James Dean suffered painful childhoods. The palpable anguish of such legendary figures is part of their unique charisma. But even knowing of the early trauma suffered by those whose ongoing emotional struggles are visible to the public, I imagined (as do so many others) that many public figures—including Laurence Olivier—had attained exceptional success, and had acquired their charismatic appeal, with the help of supportive and affirming early relationships. My close encounter with Olivier heightened my awareness of the paradoxical reality that early experiences of devastating loss, rejection, or abandonment *characteristically* fuel the drive to great achievement—not experiences of unstinting love and support.

The stories of celebrity childhoods that began to come to my attention revealed an almost infinite variety of emotional hardships. Eleanor Roosevelt's mother was harshly rejecting and died when Eleanor was only eight. Her father was an alcoholic and died when she was ten. Mikhail Baryshnikov's mother was emotionally unstable (most likely manic depressive) and committed suicide when he was eleven. Louis Armstrong was abandoned as an infant by both his parents and spent the first five years of his life in the care of his grandmother. Napoleon was sent away from his home in Corsica to attend military school in France at the age of nine. He did not see either of his parents again for five years. Virginia Woolf was a victim of sexual abuse in a family in which incest was rampant. After his parents' divorce, Charles Lindbergh was conscripted to be the caretaker and companion of his manic-depressive mother, a role that isolated him almost entirely in childhood (and well into his adulthood) from his peers.

DOI: 10.4324/9781003645757-11

I encountered one such story after another—in written as well as film biographies—stories similar in emotional tone to the description of my parents' experiences as children. And I noticed how often losses such as the ones described above caused a child to retreat from the social world around him or her and seek refuge in a more private realm of experience.

Many future writers and intellectuals, like my father (and like Freud before him), begin to read extensively at an early age. Maya Angelou retreated into books when she was sent away as a small child to live with a grandmother she had never met. Eleanor Roosevelt became an avid reader as a child. Even young Napoleon, alone in France and persecuted by his fellow students, buried himself in books of all kinds, reading most voraciously about military history

Emotionally isolated children also turn to other private avenues of self-nourishment and self-expression. Whereas Olivier began creating little theatrical dramas, Louis Armstrong learned to play the horn, Baryshnikov studied dance, and the film director Jacques Demy bought an old movie camera and taught himself to make animated films. Ansel Adams was a confirmed "darkroom monkey" by the age of fifteen.

It became clear to me that possession of highly developed skills or knowledge in adulthood is often preceded by a childhood pattern of study or practice infused with obsessive intensity—an intensity reflecting not only an inherent gratification in the activity itself, but also a need for escape from an environment that has caused intolerable distress. Baryshnikov made this connection explicit when he stated that it was because of his misery as a child that "I fell very much in love with the theater. It was my escape from family reality."

Absorption in such an activity is, on the one hand, an escape from the immediate social world; but it is also a means of connecting, on a grander scale, with other human beings. Children who turn to reading are drawn into the emotionally compelling worlds they encounter in books, where they can connect with characters who seem like safer companions than the flesh-and-blood people around them. Referring to his own childhood, James Baldwin wrote that "the people in books were more real than the people one saw every day ..."

And, of course, young musicians, dancers, and actors discover a means of connecting with others through the medium they have come to experience as their "real" emotional home, that is, the artistic realm in which they are better able to express their feelings than is possible in the context of their direct interpersonal relationships. Olivier used make-believe as a way of expressing his anguish when he began creating and acting in his own productions as a child, and Louis Armstrong expressed intense emotion through his music. A close friend once said of him that "... when Louis Armstrong wailed, he wasn't just playing a tune. He was telling the story of his life."

Absorption in a passionate interest can also be a way for a child to connect with a parent who is not otherwise emotionally available. My father's early intellectual interests were clearly stimulated by his mother's devotion to reading and to philosophy. In this mother-son relationship, the emotional issues that most deeply affected my father's sense of well-being were barred from communication. And so he bonded with his mother by studying and discussing the philosophical issues with which she was more comfortable than she could be in the realm of direct emotional intimacy.

As was the case with my father, the genius of the son or daughter often finds its outlet in an activity or art form loved by the parent, so that the shared passion contains within it a deep longing for connection with that parent. This is particularly poignant when the parent has died or succumbed to alcoholism or mental illness, leaving behind a grieving child whose commitment to the interest once shared is a desperate means of holding on to the lost object. This was a powerful factor in Baryshnikov's love of ballet—an art form his mother adored and to which she had introduced him before her tragic suicide. Amelia Earhart's father had shared with her his fascination with airplanes before he descended into alcoholism. And Charlie Chaplin's mother—herself an actress—taught him to sing songs and recite poems before she became too mentally ill to care for him and his younger brother. My father's devotion to the intellectual world was clearly a means by which he could hold on to an otherwise tenuous connection with his intellectual mother.

Reading, learning to play an instrument, dancing, acting—all of these pursuits provide children with a profound feeling of effectiveness and enhance their sense of self-worth. For children who have suffered from family circumstances beyond their control, who feel powerless to affect their own fate in the interpersonal realm, a sense of competence becomes a particularly vital source of positive self-regard. I am reminded here of my mother's reported childhood exploits—sailing off in her small dinghy "quite alone [to] try the rough parts of the lake out toward Granite Tomb." Her mastery of the elements was a desperately needed source of self-confidence in a family environment that did little to nourish self-esteem.

Fantasies of Greatness

Reading of Olivier's grandiose childhood fantasies also focused my attention on how commonly fantasies of greatness play a part in the emotional lives of children who have suffered early trauma. Children like my parents, who feel estranged from the social world around them, often survive their isolation with the help of fantasies that they, like the Ugly Duckling, are different from others in ways that will someday bring them glory. They dream that they are destined to rise above those from whom they feel alienated—to become truly extraordinary and greatly admired. This is the fantasy brought to life in fairy tales the world over in which those who feel they don't belong in the world of their peers are eventually transformed not only into beautiful swans, but also into princes and princesses, kings and queens—now in a position to bestow good fortune upon, or to reject—to forgive or not to forgive—those who have mistreated them. As in the universally gratifying tale of Cinderella, the shoe is suddenly on the other foot.

My father comforted himself in childhood with a rich fantasy life regarding his biological father, imagining him to be an artist of Danish royal blood who would someday come to embrace Dad as his special and gifted son. (This fantasy highlighted, of course, the limitations of the stepfather who could not embrace a stepson so different from himself or recognize and appreciate Dad's remarkable gifts.) My mother dreamed of pursuing a grandly adventurous career that would demonstrate her boldness, her creativity, her self-reliance, *and* her great vision. It was not until she met my father, many years later, that she found an outlet for the adventurous spirit that, in combination with his extraordinary gifts, would help her to satisfy *her* grandiose ambitions.

Olivier imagined that when he became the "greatest actor of all time," his contemptuous father and his derisive schoolmates and schoolmasters would *have* to beg his forgiveness (as in the fairy tales of old), acknowledging how badly they had misjudged and mistreated him.

Shame and Grandiosity

Andrew P. Morrison, Helen Block Lewis, and Alice Miller, among others, helped me to understand the connection between *shame*—the overwhelming feeling that one is defective, weak, and inadequate, *not good enough* as a person—and *grandiosity*—a defensive strategy for concealing feelings of inferiority behind a facade of superiority. Their perspective makes it clear why grandiose fantasy is important to the emotional survival of children whose early life circumstances have left them feeling deeply unworthy.

The psychoanalyst W.R.D. Fairbairn was one of the first to point out that when a child has been abandoned by a father who makes no effort to know or care for him; when a child's mother commits suicide or dies from other causes; when a parent is an alcoholic and/or is harshly rejecting, disapproving, or devastatingly negligent and disinterested, that child experiences the disappointment of his deepest needs as an indication that he is not deserving of love or tender care. The child's assumption is, "If I were a better child, if I were truly lovable, my parent(s) would not abandon, ignore, or reject me (that is, would not have succumbed to alcoholism or would not have died). The failure of my parent(s) to meet my most essential emotional needs is proof that there is something very wrong with me." He is filled with shame.

My father also paid special attention to the role of shame in early childhood development. He recognized that this painful feeling had been too little acknowledged in Freudian theory, which focuses on *guilt* as the emotion most pervasively responsible for psychological suffering and for psychopathology in general.

The distinction between guilt and shame is a critical one. A feeling of guilt is associated with a transgression—an action that is assumed to be deliberate and voluntary and that leads to feelings of remorse for harm done to others. Feelings of guilt rest on the assumption that one is powerful enough to have affected others adversely with one's actions. Shame, on the other hand, refers not to intentional acts but to events or situations in which one is exposed as a failure—powerless, weak, and ineffectual.

The danger associated with guilt is the threat of punishment for a transgression that has caused others harm. The danger associated with shame is the threat of abandonment and rejection because one is too deeply flawed to be worthy of acceptance by other human beings.

Dad highlighted this crucial distinction in his writing about the conflicts inherent in childhood development, but in his own efforts to understand himself, he did not use the word *shame.* For example, he spoke often about his guilt feelings toward the stepfather against whom he had rebelled, and whose last name (Homburger) he replaced with the self-invented name Erikson. I don't remember his ever acknowledging (personally or in print) the devastating effect on him of his stepfather's rejecting behavior. How deeply that must have shamed a stepson who already felt abandoned by his biological father.

When lonely and emotionally wounded children look for solace in a passionate (obsessive) interest or activity at which they find they can excel, it is natural for their heroic fantasies to center on future accomplishment in this area of special ability. This is the medium through which they imagine they will someday reveal their greatness to the world.

The Narcissistic Parent

Somewhere in the course of my early clinical training, I was introduced to Alice Miller's classic book *The Drama of the Gifted Child.* I began reading it to pass the time on a long car trip and was struck by an uncanny feeling that Alice Miller must have known my father and that this was a book *about him* and his relationship with his mother. (I have since learned that many people experience this penetrating essay as being about themselves or someone they know intimately.) I could not contain my excitement and began sharing Miller's ideas with my partner, Bob, at the end of every paragraph. Soon I was reading aloud, with frequent pauses for discussion of our personal connections with Miller's theme. The impact on both of us was profound.

Miller made it clear to me how my father's relationship to his narcissistic mother had promoted in him a profound reliance on intellect, on work, and on the need to be special (a grandiose self-image) as the most important sources of gratification and of positive self-regard. Miller explains that what we all need and long for most as children is to be loved and accepted for the small, fragile, imperfect beings that we really are. This is the kind of healthy parental acceptance that promotes the development of the child's genuine feelings of self-worth. But when a mother's (or other caretaker's) own narcissistic longings interfere with her ability to relate to the child's real needs, the child is treated as a "self object"—as someone whose reason for being is to gratify *her.* When her child reveals exceptional qualities, for example, the narcissistic mother cherishes them as a means of enhancing her own self-esteem. Her love for her child may seem intense, but it does not make the child feel loved for himself. It supports his belief that he is not worthy of love simply for being who he is, but instead must rely on his special abilities to win the care and affection of desperately needed others.

Countless superachievers have shared with my father and Olivier the experience of bonding with a mother (or father or other parental figure) who helped them to survive early tragedy and loss by making them feel intensely special. And because this parental support was so urgently needed in an otherwise desolate family environment, it *had* to be accepted as genuine love, without conscious awareness that this parent's devotion failed to satisfy the child's most basic emotional needs.

My father served as such a "self object" to his mother, who had been deeply shamed by my father's illegitimate birth and looked to him both to restore her damaged self-esteem and to fulfill the bohemian longings she had denied in herself when she married an Orthodox Jew. My father wrote about her, "I could never doubt that her ambitions for me transcended the conventions which she, nevertheless, faithfully served."

Miller's insights shed new light on the pervasive sadness I had always felt in my father—a sadness that persisted despite his enormous success. I had, until then, imagined that his underlying depression related primarily to his abandonment by an unidentified father. I now understood that in addition to this loss, Dad had been made to feel that it was his gifts that had earned him a special place in his mother's heart, and that it was his talent on which he must continue to rely to secure love and attention from those closest to him. I was overwhelmed with recognition.

Olivier always knew that as much as his mother adored him, to make her happy, he must be a *star.* And Picasso's mother proclaimed her quintessentially narcissistic expectations of her son when she told him, "If you become a soldier, you'll be a general. If you become a priest, you'll end up the Pope!" Is it any wonder that Picasso entitled an early self-portrait *Yo el Rey* ("I the King")—repeated three times for emphasis?

But the truly awesome influence of a parent's narcissistic needs could not be better illustrated than by the story of Frank Lloyd Wright, whose choice of profession was decided for him by his mother before he was born. During her pregnancy, Wright's mother felt certain that she would have a son who was not only destined for greatness but was also destined for greatness *as an architect.* His career was propelled and guided from the moment of his birth by his mother's will.

A narcissistic parent plays a critical role in encouraging not only the development of a child's talent, but also his or her reliance on that talent as a source of self-esteem. Responding to their parents' narcissistic needs, children can come to believe that it is only their special gifts that can be counted upon to secure care and affection from people important to their survival—that they are not worthy of love for simply being themselves. That being the case, they must then work ceaselessly to impress the world with their talent. The dreaded alternative is to be completely ignored, left abandoned, and alone.

At the same time, when a child has experienced his or her power to gratify a parent's desires and to secure the intense interest of this essential person through the demonstration of special ability, his or her sense of grandiosity is inevitably inflated. There is no better fuel for grandiose ambition than the experience of being very special to a narcissistically needy parent. It was astounding to me to discover how often such a parent lurks behind the scenes in the lives of superachievers.

When Work Is More Than Just Work

When early experiences have encouraged a child to retreat from the wider social world into a passionate and obsessive personal interest, that child often becomes an adult who is preoccupied with work. For example, my father didn't really live in the same world as the rest of us. He lived in a special universe that he referred to as "my work," the physical locus of which was his study. From there he visited us for events like dinner or a family outing (or in the Orinda days, a swim); but like anyone visiting from another universe, he found family life rather alien and was awkward and uncomfortable among us.

Of course, there *was* a cultural difference between my father and the rest of us. He had grown up in Germany, so the language and the norms of our twentieth-century American household were literally foreign to him, whereas my Canadian-American mother was completely at home with both. But that was not the ultimate basis for Dad's insecurity as a member of the family. He didn't really know how to engage with people comfortably when the content of the interaction was unrelated to his work or, more broadly, to intellectual issues that dovetailed with his work. Within the family as a social unit, he was frequently at a loss.

It is not hard to understand why a person like my father often continues to be preoccupied as an adult with the interest or activity that sustained him in childhood. It was in the pursuit of his artistic and intellectual interests that he experienced himself in the most positive light, where he felt in touch with an *ideal self* that represented all that he most wanted to be. The ideal self is the antithesis, in important respects, of the ways in which a person feels himself to be most deeply flawed. And when a passionate interest connects a person with his most positive self-image, diminishing his sense of personal defectiveness, it becomes his emotional home—the place where he is happiest and most alive and at ease.

Laurence Olivier confessed to a perpetual restlessness when he was not engaged in some way with the theater. "I am filled with unease," he wrote, "if I am doing anything other than working. Work is life for me, it is the only point in life." Albert Einstein was famously obsessed with his work, and there is good evidence that most of the greatest thinkers in human history have been equally so. In his book *Greatness,* Dean Keith Simonton suggests that it is, in fact, a "monomaniacal preoccupation" with work that distinguishes the greatest figures in every field of human endeavor. "It takes work," he declares, "to become a renowned genius. These individuals are driven by huge motivational forces that far eclipse the impetus behind less accomplished colleagues."

For those who have embraced a passionate interest early in life and have made the pursuit of that interest the *point* of their life, work is not simply work. It is a universe within which the individual feels safer, more comfortable, and more purposeful than he does in the world of intimate personal relationships. For such a person, the moments of greatest intimacy occur in the sharing of their work—not only with an audience, but also with colleagues and students who are dedicated to the same passionate pursuits or with admirers who are deeply touched by the work. As awkward as he might feel in social situations where ideas were not the focus of attention, my father became strikingly engaged, animated, and self-confident any time he was called upon to discuss ideas, especially his own. There was nothing he enjoyed more than giving a personal tour of *his* universe. As a result, those for whom he served as teacher, supervisor, or mentor felt very intimately connected with him.

Olivier confessed to an extreme lack of comfort with social situations, lamenting that parties had "literally made me feel ill, even to the extent of swooning away and having to be half-carried from the room." Like many performers, he felt more at ease, more powerful, more excited and alive when he was on the stage than when he was off. Similarly, the British actress Elaine Paige has said about performing, "I think I'm at my most happy when I'm on stage. I feel relaxed and at ease and in control. Acting … gives me a license to be more powerful and interesting than I could ever possibly be in real life." Tennessee Williams wrote that "it is only in his work that an artist can find reality and satisfaction, for the actual world is less intense than the world of his invention and consequently his life, without recourse to violent disorder, does not seem very substantial."

The Celebrity and the Public

Work is more than just work, in another profound sense, for the person who has survived the assaults of childhood with the help of fantasies of future greatness. A person who longs for celebrity may hope that a parent who has not shown sufficient interest will be impressed by the achievement of fame and will come to appreciate his or her child more. I know that my mother hoped her marriage to an up-and-coming intellectual superstar would finally win her the approval of her harshly critical mother. My father, of course, entertained the fantasy that his real father might learn of his renown and want to know his famous son. James Dean was desperately disappointed that his stardom failed to win the interest and approval of the father who had abandoned him in childhood.

On the other hand, when a parent has encouraged the child's reliance on grandiose fantasy, the public can be experienced as an extension of that parent. Both Olivier and Baryshnikov lost, early in childhood, the mother who had cherished and encouraged their talent. So for them, the adulation of an audience provided (or continues to provide) a powerful connection with the lost love object.

In a more general sense, however, the public itself becomes the object of the longing for parental love. And it often seems to the person seeking fame that it is only the recognition and admiration of a vast number of people that can fill the void left by parental neglect. The psychoanalyst Otto Fenichel has suggested that the love of the audience "is needed in the same way as milk and affection are needed by the infant."

It is the public (an audience), after all, that offers any human being—but especially those in a state of profound need—the most exhilarating form of narcissistic gratification: the intense adulation of people who experience one as being very special. Perhaps the excited adoration of an audience is the closest any of us can come to reexperiencing in adulthood—or experiencing for the first time—the passionate love of a mother who is crazy about her baby, and perceives him or her to be the most important being in the world. Jerry Lewis once acknowledged that the applause of an audience sounds to him like "Good baby, good baby." And Eartha Kitt said in an interview, "I was an orphan until the public, thank God, adopted me."

Although I did not understand the importance to my parents of being adored and admired by the outside world, I was aware, even as a child, that the presence of any audience—even admiring friends—made them feel better about themselves, more vital, warm, and alive than they felt in the privacy of the family home.

My parents needed continuous confirmation of the idealized (grandiose) self-image that had helped them survive childhood emotionally intact. And both succeeded (even before my father became famous) in getting that affirmation from admiring friends and even from the children of friends. But their *own* children could not provide such unwavering adulation. Children are inevitably ambivalent toward their parents—needing to express anger and resentment as well as love and gratitude for the ways in which their dependency needs are (or are not) met. When parents themselves feel unworthy of love, it is difficult for them to tolerate their children's ambivalence, experiencing it as a confirmation of their personal inadequacies rather than as a normal part of the parent-child relationship. This was a source of unending strain in my relationship with my parents. As deeply as I loved both of them, my love (and that of my brothers) failed to affirm them in the way they needed most.

I suspect that Joan Crawford's infamous rage toward her children reflected (in a *far* more extreme way) just such an inability to believe in their love for her—no matter how hard they tried to show her that she meant everything to them. Only the wholehearted adulation of the larger world could provide Crawford with relief from the self-hatred that she saw reflected in the eyes of her children—though, paradoxically, it was they who loved her the most.

The need for relief from such inner demons often drives the pursuit of fame, and it interferes, at the same time, with the ability of those who need public adulation to connect as intensely with the people close to them as they do with their admirers. The grandiose self (or ideal self) is, of course, a fragile internal structure. It might be defined as a self-image that is perfect and infallible in all the ways the person was made to feel, as a child, that he or she was *not.*

The challenge of intimate personal relationships is that they require a willingness to accept in oneself and to reveal to others one's "flaws," both real and imagined. To be capable of genuine intimacy, one must feel acceptable to others *in spite of* being flawed, so that one's defenses can gradually be let down and more of the self revealed. When a person feels compelled to hide behind the mask of an ideal self, the demands of intimacy can seem very threatening indeed. It may feel safer to court the public, relying on an idealized public image as a safeguard against potentially devastating self-exposure.

John Updike said in a recent interview, "This need for another self, a superior, a public self is, I guess, very deep for me.... Maybe I wasn't satisfied with the self I had. I wanted to construct a better one."

It took me many years to begin to understand the connection between my father's public image as the quintessential parent and provider of emotional nourishment to the young, and the awkward, insecure father of my private experience. But it gradually became clear to me that there is *always* such a paradoxical relationship between an idealized public image (a reflection of the ideal self) and the person as he experiences himself, and is experienced by others, in the private realm. Such is the paradoxical nature of grandiose images. The more spectacular they are, the greater the intensity of the shame and self-contempt they are being called upon to conceal.

...

These insights about my father's relationship to his work, to his public, and to his idealized public image have all helped me to come to terms with my personal experience of him. They have helped me understand why—even though I always felt Dad loved me—he never seemed as fully present in his interactions with me as he was when talking with people who saw him as *Erik Erikson.* He could engage more deeply with Mom, who was not only a partner in his work but also a recipient of emotional sustenance from his fame. To her, he *was Erik Erikson* as well as the insecure husband who needed so much care and support. And when Kai grew up to become an eminent intellectual (a sociologist) in his own right, he and Dad could talk for hours about their work. They even wrote and talked publicly together.

Kai could be close to Dad as a fellow intellectual, but I resented Dad's primary commitment to his work and rebelled against the competition. And when you cannot (or *will* not) relate to a superachiever through his work, you are forever consigned to living in a different universe. Only now, as I find myself increasingly able to appreciate and embrace the richness of my father's special world, can I enjoy a deeper and more gratifying sense of connection with him.

Chapter 11

Going Public Myself

Two years after I had begun analytic training, as my perspective on the psychological nature of fame was developing, I offered to present my ideas to my colleagues at the counseling center where I was on staff. The situation was paradoxical. On the one hand, I had begun to feel more like my father in my new conviction that my ideas were worth sharing with others. Yet what had made it safe enough for me to enjoy this identification with him was the belief that I was quite different from him (and Mother) in my less desperate need for public affirmation as a source of self-esteem. The more clearly I understood what had driven my parents to rely so heavily on the gratification of fame, the safer I felt allowing myself to seek some of the rewards of professional recognition without fearing that I would succumb to the family addiction.

And I had a perspective that I wanted very much to share. I had been uncomfortable for years with the kinds of assumptions people made about my experience as the daughter of a famous man—assumptions about how uniquely affirming and glamorous my family life must have been, and how lucky I was to have been born with the silver spoon of fame in my mouth. I wanted to share my real experience with some of the people who mattered most to me. I thought there was value in it for them, too, since in idealizing my father (as well as other celebrities), they seemed to be undervaluing themselves and their own accomplishments. They were imagining that someone else more fortunate than they were had all the blessings they wished for in their own lives: worldwide renown and the ultimate sense of accomplishment and of self-acceptance that such celebrity must surely bring. I wanted to tell them what a mixed blessing I had discovered fame to be.

But I was also anxious about this first presentation to my colleagues. For years, I had wondered (as had some of those closest to me) whether my perspective on fame was simply a defensive device used to express anger toward my fame-obsessed parents. It was partly that, of course. And I knew that some who heard these ideas would experience them as simply an attack on the edifice of my father's fame. I knew from long years of experience that many people cared far more about preserving their idealized image of my father than about hearing my perspective on his fame. I would be inviting harsh criticism, and it terrified me.

DOI: 10.4324/9781003645757-12

Fame Does Not Heal

It appeared to their admirers that my parents had transcended the greatest hardships of life and had been healed and made whole by the achievement of renown. Many believed that what my parents had achieved was the most a person could possibly hope for in life. And, of course, my parents did enjoy many advantages and pleasures as a result of Dad's celebrity. But what was concealed behind their glowing public image was a sad reality: that fame had *not* healed their early childhood wounds. This is where the psychology of human beings differs profoundly from the psychology of fairy-tale heroes.

Consider the story of Snow White. Her mother dies when she is born. When she is seven, her stepmother, envious of her budding beauty, commands a huntsman to kill her. The huntsman reneges, and the enraged stepmother tries to do the job herself with a poison apple. Fortunately, the kiss of a handsome prince reverses the effects of the poison before it is too late. Snow White and the prince marry and live happily ever after. Remarkably, the kiss of the prince has restored Snow White's *mental* as well as her physical health. The murderous hatred of her stepmother (the only mother she has ever known) has caused no lasting damage to her trust in others, her self-esteem, or her capacity to love.

For Cinderella, too, happiness lies ahead. The love of her prince will erase the effects of her childhood loss and abuse. For human beings, however, recovery from early trauma is more difficult. We would like to think that fame, like the kiss of the fairy-tale prince, can magically heal our wounded idols. But in real life the kiss of a prince offers few tangible health benefits, and celebrity is a very imperfect cure.

What the love of the public cannot do is affirm the famous in the way that they, and, indeed, all of us, most need to be affirmed—for being *ourselves,* in all our glory and in all our flawed vulnerability. As much as it might seem that certain public figures *are* idolized for being "just themselves," their personal qualities are revealed to the public only through the prism of an idealized image that distorts the truth, often in the very paradoxical way I have described above. What are really adored are the gifts of the celebrity and his or her public persona, not the person behind the public mask. And no one is more aware of this than the object of the adulation.

Writing about the "catastrophe" of his success, Tennessee Williams lamented: "You know … that the public Somebody you are when you 'have a name' is a fiction created with mirrors and that the only somebody worth being is the solitary and unseen you that existed from your first breath …. "

That is why the devotion of the public could not be experienced by my father as acclaim for himself as a *person.* And it was not, therefore, a source of genuine self-esteem. Such adulation could not be internalized by him in the way that the early love of parents is incorporated into—and becomes a lasting part of—a child's psyche, providing a foundation for genuine self-acceptance.

Fame is more like a psychological addiction: an emotional dependence on a type of experience needed to ward off depression and feelings of emptiness. That experience cannot permanently dispel an underlying dysphoria, but can only relieve it temporarily. And once such relief has been savored, it enhances the craving for more of the commodity that can banish emotional pain.

Fame did offer my father moments of great exhilaration when his grandiose sense of self was powerfully affirmed. But those moments were, by nature, fleeting, and the exhilaration short-lived. Even the most enthusiastic audiences eventually stop applauding and go home. Popular excitement about the most glorious achievements diminishes with the passing of time. And since these intensely affirming experiences cannot be internalized in a way that permanently enhances the celebrity's sense of himself or herself, they do not satisfy the appetite for approval. Rather, they feed that appetite and deepen the longing for more such intense adulation.

When you have experienced being the center of the universe, the loss of that position can feel like a profound abandonment. It is no surprise that so many rock stars, worshiped as gods while on the stage, feel bereft when the concert is over and turn to promiscuous sex and drugs to fill the emotional void. My father, too, seemed to feel let down after important public events where he was the object of excited attention. It was difficult for him to readjust to life without that heightened affirmation of his importance to others—to make do with the more mundane gratifications of everyday living and relating. He would be restless and a bit depressed. He would watch eagerly for the mailman, who just might bring some affirming message from the outside world.

Not only is public acclaim addictive, resulting in painful symptoms of withdrawal when one is no longer in the limelight, but there is a hidden cost to being known widely through the prism of a public image—"a fiction created with mirrors," in the words of Tennessee Williams. When you are perceived by the public to be more glamorous, more powerful, more confident, more *perfect* than any mortal can truly be or feel, the result is bound to be a sense of personal fraudulence. Your human imperfections seem the more shameful in contrast to the idealized version of yourself that has been projected onto the public screen. And, of course, you live in dread of exposure.

My father's idealized image as a father figure increased his sense of shame that he could not be the kind of parent he so wanted to be to his own children. It actually made him feel *more* inadequate in the realm where it was assumed he would be uniquely competent. In fact, my father's public image placed a burden on all of us, seeming to require that we be something more than we experienced ourselves as being. I am reminded of my mother's lament that she could not talk to her dearest friend about a family crisis because of "Erik's reputation." We *all* lived with the sense that there were family secrets we needed to hide: that our father was not as infallible as he appeared in the public light; that our family was not as perfect as the family of a world-famous psychoanalyst ought to be; and that none of us (his children) were as perfect as we surely should be given our illustrious parentage. We all felt compelled to sustain a family image consistent with our father's reputation. And, in fact, our behavior *was* important to the preservation of Dad's image. He could not disguise his inevitable concern that we reflect well on him.

But as burdensome as an idealized image can be to its bearer (and often to that person's closest of kin), it is still not as heavy as the knowledge that the love and admiration of the public rests on one's ability to perform or to produce at a consistently superior level. We tend to believe that people who have achieved fame have arrived at a place of security and completeness where fame means no longer needing to prove themselves. But the truth is quite the opposite. Every accomplishment experienced by the celebrity as a validation of his or her special gifts also represents a challenge: "Will I be able to do it again? Will my next achievement be as well received as my last? What if I lose my gift?" Those held in the highest public esteem cannot help but fear that their awe-inspiring talents might suddenly fail them, resulting in a catastrophic fall from grace.

As driven as Dad was while writing his first book, *Childhood and Society*; he had less to lose during this creative process than he had while writing his subsequent books. As his career progressed, there was no escaping the intense pressure to maintain the level of excellence he had once achieved. Laurence Olivier acknowledged his constant anxiety that someone watching him perform for the first time might ask, "What is all the fuss about?" His fear of not living up to his reputation culminated in a prolonged bout with stage fright that nearly forced his premature retirement from acting.

Vulnerability to Criticism

And there is still another emotional burden that celebrities must bear, one seldom recognized by those who idealize fame. Public acclaim *always* means negative as well as positive recognition. We know and understand, in retrospect, that all the greatest achievements of the human race have been met with contempt and outrage by many who first passed judgment on them. The greatest pioneers of human history have all been reviled as well as celebrated. (Consider the public condemnation that greeted the ideas of Galileo, Darwin, or Freud.)

It is not just resistance to innovation that evokes public condemnation of the renowned. The most gifted among us are naturally held to a higher standard and their accomplishments more harshly judged. Likewise, those blessed with originality and charisma are natural targets of criticism as well as adoration just by virtue of the fact that they evoke intense feelings in others through their works, their performances, or their public personalities. Such intense feelings inevitably run the gamut from love to disapproval, if not outright hatred. In fact, the more intense the public adoration of a celebrity, the more intense will be his or her *disfavor* in the eyes of some. And this disfavor becomes a constant part of his or her awareness.

In their quest for cosmic approval, the famous become enormous targets for the barbs of public criticism, and they are, at the same time, exceptionally vulnerable to those barbs. I have described how much my father suffered over the criticism directed at him in the 1970s. The shelter of an idealized self-image is an imperfect shelter indeed. Not only is a grandiose sense of self inherently fragile, but it also requires the constant support of others who, out of their own need, help to maintain the idealization. When an observer has reason to question the grandiose image rather than accept it at face value—as when Dorothy challenges the formidable facade of the Wizard of Oz, or when the child exposes the emperor's pretensions in the story of the emperor's new clothes—the true fragility of such a facade is instantly revealed, illustrating the ease with which any grandiose image can be penetrated by anyone who dares to look behind it.

The tragic irony of this defense is that although the approval of the vast majority is *not* experienced as being about the real self, criticism *is* experienced as being about the real self behind the public persona. Criticism penetrates the mask, making one feel "found out"—exposed in all one's self-perceived defectiveness. No amount of public adoration can inoculate the narcissistically vulnerable against the pain of inevitable disapproval—even from the most insignificant quarter.

The Disappointment of Grandiose Ambition

As hard as it may be for the admirers of the superambitious to imagine, grandiose ambition is never truly satisfied. The ultimate goal of the grandiose self is, after all, to be perfect—beyond criticism and beyond competition, to be "the best," to be "the greatest of all time." The more limited rewards of renown are inevitably a disappointment.

This ultimate pitfall of fame came to my attention during the years after my father's book *Ghandi's Truth* was published in 1969, and my parents talked quietly about the possibility of a Nobel Prize. *Ghandi's Truth* had already won a Pulitzer Prize and the National Book Award. But these profound expressions of recognition were not enough. Their hearts were set on the highest prize of all, and it was a letdown that it was never bestowed upon Dad.

In a similar vein, Woody Allen has confessed that he did not get what he really wanted either: "I had grandiose plans for myself when I started. And I have not lived up to them. I've done some things that are perfectly nice. But I had a much grander conception of where I should end up in the artistic firmament." Allen reflects on what might have brought him more profound satisfaction with his work: "I regret that my muse was a comic muse and not a dramatic muse. I would rather have had the gifts of Eugene O'Neill or Tennessee Williams than the gifts I got. I'm not kvetching. I'm glad I got any gifts at all. But I would like to do something great."

Leonard Bernstein's children have also revealed the sense of disappointment that haunted their father toward the end of his career, when he despaired that his music was not good enough; that he was not "taken seriously" as a composer. He had wanted to be Gustav Mahler No. 2. I believe my father wanted to be another Freud.

The envy felt by the exceptionally gifted for the talents and achievements of others reflects their disappointment that no amount of success ever makes a person feel that he or she has *made it*—has arrived safely in the kingdom of the great. Those who have experienced this disappointment in relation to their own grandiose fantasies seem to imagine that their role models (Eugene O'Neill, Tennessee Williams, Mahler, or Freud) *do* reside safely in that kingdom. The assumption is that those others *must* feel what the enviers don't: a profound sense of satisfaction with what they have accomplished, a sense of importance in the "firmament."

My father experienced something similar toward the end of his career: a disappointment with what he had achieved and an envy of others who seemed to be reaping a kind of reward that, for all his fame, he had not attained. He was well aware that his contemporary, the psychoanalyst Heinz Kohut, had acquired a significant following in the field and had founded a new school of psychoanalysis referred to as "self psychology" Dad's close friend Margaret Brenman-Gibson reports that he once said to her, "All I hear these days is self psychology. Well, Margaret, what history will say is that Erikson tried, but Kohut made it." Brenman-Gibson assured him he was "nuts" and that his work was important on an entirely different level from Kohut's, but Dad "appeared to be unpersuaded."

Enough Is Never Enough

Retirement is the last, and perhaps the greatest, narcissistic blow to anyone who has relied on work and public acclaim as a primary source of self-esteem and of meaning in life. Laurence Olivier retired in his mid-seventies, when health problems made it impossible for him to continue to act. And he was soon overwhelmed with the depression and anxiety that had haunted him throughout his life whenever he was not working. The result was a continual series of physical infirmities that plagued his last years.

At the end of a celebrated life, there is never a moment when enough has been accomplished, and the celebrity can retire with a well-earned sense of pride and fulfillment. It would be a simpler matter if the self-esteem of the famous rested on what they have already accomplished. But what they have already accomplished is rarely experienced by them as being good enough. And so, of course, to stop producing or accomplishing represents the end of hope that one's grandiose ambitions will ever be fulfilled. As a result, the retirement of the most accomplished is rarely experienced as an opportunity to bask in the successes of the past. It represents, instead, the end of opportunity to ever get it right—to do something truly *great*, to live up to one's real potential and to feel satisfied with oneself at last. Because no one ever feels they have made it to the top, there is never a good time to rest.

And, of course, the appetite for public adoration and applause is never sated. Those who have relied on public acclaim as a source of relief from inner demons find themselves alone with those demons when they are no longer in the limelight. Loved ones may be able to make life easier in the final years; but for the most part, intimate relationships do not stave off the feelings of unworthiness and depression that characteristically lurk behind the most grandiose facades. To those who have needed applause the most, its cessation feels like a terrible abandonment.

...

The response to my first lecture about fame was transforming for me. My insights about the psychological realities of being famous, which had helped me so much to differentiate from my parents, aroused excited interest in my colleagues. I was not made to feel like a vengeful daughter, but rather like someone whose personal experience had become a source of useful and important ideas.

What surprised me most, I think, was that others at that lecture identified with me, describing their own experience of parents whose special status in a community or whose prestigious occupation invited idealization by those around them. It became clear that my experience of my father's fame was not nearly as unique as I had imagined, but was only different in degree from the experiences of many others whose parents also struggled in private with their demons, while maintaining an idealized image to conceal their shame.

This lecture to my colleagues was the first of a number I was to give over the next few years as my thoughts about fame developed and expanded. I had found a level of self (and family) revelation that was comfortable enough for me, despite the emotional repercussions that followed each time I talked about my own and my parents' demons. I often dreamed, after these lectures, that I was naked and exposed in some public setting. But the response to my ideas from other psychotherapists and psychoanalysts was consistently affirming. I had found a new way to tame my personal monsters—not only by analyzing them and talking about them in private, but also by speaking about them publicly, and finding my insights meaningful to others.

That didn't mean, though, that I was ready to broadcast my views on a scale that would bring them to my mother's attention. When my father died in 1994, I spoke at his memorial service, gently acknowledging my struggle with his fame and with the idealized image of him that had haunted our father-daughter relationship. I could not say good-bye to my father without expressing this sense of loss along with my enduring feelings of love for him. But I worried about how my words would sound to my grieving mother. These were not the kinds of truths that any of us generally expressed in her presence. In the end, I was not sure whether she even heard my talk. The ceremony may have been a blur to her in her state of mourning; she never said a word to me about my remarks on that occasion.

Mom's Last Years

Dad had retired almost completely from the world around him by the time of his death. In his last years he seemed serene in an inner world, responding with a smile when he recognized his wife and children, but it was no longer clear that he knew who most of us really were. He muttered a few words, but those were mostly to himself. I was deeply touched on one visit to Dad when a flash of pleasure crossed his face as I entered the room, and he said faintly to himself, *Meine Tochter* ("my daughter" in his native tongue).

Mother had seen to it, of course, that Dad's physical care was excellent, and he lived to the age of ninety-two. But though she cherished the moments when he emerged briefly from his private reverie to indicate his pleasure at seeing her, she missed his company terribly and was sometimes overwhelmed with sadness at having to make a life for herself alone.

A full-page photograph of my parents that had appeared in the *Boston Globe* in 1987 (seven years before Dad's death) had already revealed both the faraway look in my father's eyes that was characteristic by that time and the profound grief that sometimes revealed itself—even then—in Mother's lovely face. When this photograph appeared, I was shocked by the depth of her sadness and wondered, "Isn't it obvious to *everyone*?" Yet no one seemed to see past the idealization of my parents to notice how things really were, or knew what to say to me if they *did* notice. The reactions to that article were the usual: "Your parents are *so* distinguished looking." And the accompanying article ("Partners for Life") described the vital collaboration between my parents that the author imagined was still going strong.

Mother did everything possible to sustain this deception. For as long as she could, she publicly denied Dad's intellectual decline, celebrating—and often exaggerating—every sign on his part that he understood what visitors said to him. Interviews were given in which Dad sat silently while Mother did all the talking, referring to him as though he were still actively engaged with her in the furthering of his own ideas. I remember a Christmas newsletter in the late 1980s that reported that "Erik continues to work on 'The Galilean Sayings'"—a sad distortion of the truth, which was that Dad was barely in communication with the outside world at all. What underlay that distortion was, of course, Mother's dread of being abandoned by the world should it become known that her link with greatness was no longer viable.

As deeply loved and admired as my mother was by people all over the country (and in other parts of the world as well), she was terrified that friends would abandon her once Dad was no longer an active part of her life. And she feared, too, that Dad's work would not be remembered or sufficiently honored once his productivity had stopped. She devoted herself to projects that she thought would sustain his memory, working obsessively, for example, to find a publisher for a journal Dad had kept as a young man, though few who saw it felt it was reflective of Dad's later brilliance. Mom anticipated not only her own loss of importance in the world, but his as well. She after all, had been profoundly abandoned as a child, and such early traumas can return to haunt the very elderly, for whom abandonment and neglect is always the ultimate fear.

Despite this terror, though, Mother remained physically and intellectually vital into her nineties and enjoyed talking and writing about her own ideas. As worried as she was that Dad's work would be neglected, she also experienced this time as an opportunity to focus on her own writing. She clearly hoped to become more widely recognized, now, for her *own* considerable gifts. She wrote several chapters about the aging process that were published as an addendum to Dad's book *The Life Cycle Completed* in 1997. But the response was not what she longed for—that her work would engender the kind of enthusiasm and excitement that had greeted Dad's writing many years before. In her most cherished fantasies, people would say, "My God, she was *always* just as smart as he was, and now she should be honored as his equal." But her own chapters in *Life Cycle* did not win her that sort of acclaim, and the revised edition did not sell very well.

Her lack of success as a writer, relative to my father's *enormous* success, was the great disappointment of my mother's professional life. I often wonder whether she dedicated herself, ultimately, to the written word because it was the commodity most highly valued in the intellectual world in which she found herself as Dad's wife. Given the enormity of her other talents—particularly her craftsmanship as a jeweler (as demonstrated by the superb, award-winning jewelry she made in the 1940s and 1950s)—I sometimes feel sad that she did not continue to reap the rewards that this medium so generously offered her.

During the last years of Mother's life, while I was in psychoanalytic training, we had weekly telephone conversations in which she asked my advice on matters that troubled her, or reported accomplishments of which she felt proud. Though she referred to me often as her "therapist," and spoke of how helpful I was to her, she *never* followed my advice, nor had she ever done so in the course of our adult relationship. I urged her, for example, to let go of her anxiety about Dad's image and about her own writing—both sources of continued anguish for her—assuring her that she and Dad had already established themselves firmly on this planet. But continuing to achieve was her lifeline, and no amount of daughterly reassurance could temper the urgency of that need.

My Dilemma

Still, I found myself on the horns of a dilemma. I felt a growing desire to write about my experience of family life and fame—something I knew would be painful for Mother. My longing to claim my own professional authority emerged at just the moment when Mother felt that she was losing hers. She lived in fear that Dad's idealized reputation would diminish with his death just when I was prepared to challenge *all* idealized images. This was not the time to confront, publicly, Mother's need for celebrity *or* her limited understanding of the emotional forces that had propelled her toward the celebrated life. I knew I would have to wait.

As it happened, an important biography of my parents was being prepared at this time by the historian Lawrence Friedman. Friedman had talked to innumerable family friends (as well as to all of the Erikson family members) in the course of his biographical research, and one such friend had told him the story of Neil, the child with Down syndrome who had never been brought home to live with the Erikson family. This piece of information not only took Friedman by surprise, but it also became a focal point of his further research and of his eventual book *Identity's Architect: A Biography of Erik H. Erikson.*

I knew from Larry's interviews with me that his biography of my parents would be candid and revealing, and that the crisis of Neil's birth would be treated extensively. I myself had never talked publicly about Neil, and even *I* winced at the idea that this deeply painful wound was to be publicly probed. I was, of course, concerned about how this revelation would affect Mother, even though she had shared with Larry her own memories of those long-ago events. The fact was that few people who had been part of my parents' life since they'd left California in 1950 knew *anything* about Neil. Most of Mother's closest friends were not aware that he had ever existed, so the book could be expected to shock many who felt they knew my parents well. (A number of Mother's close friends *did* express astonishment to me after Larry's book was published.)

But Mother did not live to see the publication of this biography. She died in 1997 at the age of ninety-four. Loyal family friends had continued to call and visit her up until the time she died, still enjoying her vitality, her generous and lively spirit, and her scarcely diminished clarity of thought. This continued affection on the part of so many longtime friends—as well as some new and adoring ones—was vitally important to her. As much as she cherished family visits—and it was always clear that she did—I never knew her to tell someone who called or who dropped by unexpectedly, "I can't talk (or visit) right now because my children/ grandchildren are here." The need for affirmation from the outside world was as strong in her later years as it had been early in our childhoods.

Whether my fears were exaggerated or not, I was relieved that Mother would not have to deal with the public response to Friedman's biography. And soon after her death, I began to feel twice liberated in my own need to write about our family life. I could no longer cause her pain, and there were no more family secrets to hide. Larry had told them all. I was now free to recount *my* experience, and my personal understanding of it—not so much to report what had happened as to explain it from my personal perspective.

It was not long after the publication of *Identity's Architect* that I was invited to give a colloquium at the analytic institute where I had, by then, completed my training. This was my most important lecture to date, the audience being made up of the faculty members who had been my teachers and mentors, students who had trained before and with me in this analytic program, and some close friends whom I had asked to come and share what felt like an official "coming out" for me. I worked hard to organize the ideas that I would share for the first time with the people whose opinion meant the most to me, and the evening was one of the most exciting and gratifying of my life. It confirmed that my perspective on fame was personally meaningful to others, and that the theoretical issues I had raised were considered valid and important by the people who had taught me psychoanalytic theory. It was suggested that I publish the paper I presented that night, and it was accepted a few months later by the *Atlantic Monthly*; to appear under the heading "Fame: The Power and Cost of a Fantasy." I had, indeed, gone public.

Chapter 12

The Eye of the Beholder

The responses to my *Atlantic Monthly* article were the first I had gotten from the public at large, and they were both affirming and disconcerting. There were letters of gratitude from many who had had family experiences similar to mine and appreciated my acknowledging my struggle with my father's fame. There were thoughtful reactions to some of the ideas about the relationship between early trauma and high achievement, with suggestions regarding books or articles that might be of interest to me. And there were those who made it clear that they did *not* appreciate the portrayal of my father as a less-than-perfect human being, and would have preferred that I had kept my personal experience to myself.

The most extreme reactions were from people who had known and adored my parents. In one instance, it was suggested that I hated both Mom and Dad, and in another that I was trying to "settle a score" with them. One old family friend thought that I had "embarrassed" myself in writing the article, and another was "sorry you felt you had to do that." There was a shaming quality to these reprimands. The implication was that I was a bad daughter whose mission was to tarnish my father's image and to take away from others the blessings my father had bestowed on them.

These reactions evoked early feelings of shame about the inappropriateness of expressing my feelings and of affirming my own experience at the expense of my parents' idealized image. It was clear there would be no panacea in sharing my personal story. It might diminish the extent to which I felt eclipsed by my father's fame, but it would provide no safety from the old familiar threats to my self-esteem.

I encountered just such a threat when I was invited, soon after the publication of the *Atlantic Monthly* article, to speak at a meeting of psychoanalysts in New York City. It was suggested that I bring a videotape of my father to play for a few minutes to give those attending a glimpse of what he was like in person. I happened to have a tape of my father being interviewed—in the prime of his life and career—and brought it along, as requested. The talk was going well, I thought. The group was small but engaged and showed a lively interest in my ideas. But when I began to play the tape of my father, the room became quiet and attentive in a whole different way. I could feel Dad's magic—his charisma—capture this audience, and it was immediately clear that no one was going to want this tape to end. I knew that the recorded interview with my father continued for a full hour, and I felt a sense

DOI: 10.4324/9781003645757-13

of panic that my talk was suddenly over, and the evening now belonged to *him.* I felt obliterated, as I had so many times before in my life, and wished—for just a moment—that I had never set myself up for this public humiliation.

The tape *did* eventually get turned off, and I resumed my talk without confessing to those present what I had just experienced. Since then, I have often wished that I *had* told them of my feelings at that moment. After all, my brief sense of being eclipsed is at the very heart of my perspective on the power of fame and its potential effect on all of us.

The event also confronted me once again with the mystery of my father's charisma. What was it that made his image on the screen so compelling? In the *Atlantic Monthly* article, I had talked about the universal human need to believe in idealized images and heroic figures, citing the ideas of the anthropologist/philosopher Ernest Becker in his brilliant book *The Denial of Death.* Becker makes the profound observation that even those members of our species to whom we ascribe the most magical powers are, in reality, just *"Homo sapiens,* standard vintage," practically indistinguishable from the rest of us except for *the aura we project onto them* in order to meet our own needs. Our idealization of them arises more out of our need to worship than out of qualities that truly distinguish them from ourselves.

We *must* have heroes, Becker explains, because the real world is simply too terrible for us to face without them. We are born small and helpless and continue all our lives to feel terrifyingly vulnerable, having little control over the forces of nature or of life and death, and often powerless to affect our fate. And, most frightening of all, we know that we are going to die. We are the only species burdened with this unbearable knowledge. We need people among us who seem less helpless than ourselves, people who seem to be possessed of superhuman strengths, abilities, and virtues that make us feel less vulnerable and less inadequate *as a species* and enhance our precarious status in the cosmos.

It is when we are the smallest and most helpless of all, when we are children, that we first stake our lives on the belief that grown-ups—and most important, our parents—have the power to protect us from the destructive forces of the universe. Childhood without that illusion is psychologically intolerable, and so, as children, we sacrifice our sense of reality whenever we must to preserve the belief that our parents are capable of keeping us safe from harm. This willingness to distort reality to preserve an idealized image of our caretakers follows us into adulthood.

My father radiated a compassionate paternal authority that made him the most natural of transference figures. It was Freud who first used the term *transference* to describe the way in which we transfer our childlike feelings of dependency from parents to a physician or other authority figure, exaggerating the powers of such individuals as we once exaggerated those of our original caretakers, to make ourselves feel better protected. In the transference we ascribe extra powers to others in whom we need to believe. The psychoanalyst Irving Yalom has labeled this the "ultimate rescuer defense," the human tendency "to manufacture a godlike figure and then to bask in the illusion of safety emanating from our creation." And Erich Fromm has written eloquently about the human tendency to escape from "freedom," the realization of our own separateness and individuality, by fusing ourselves with somebody or something outside of ourselves in order to acquire from them the strength we believe we lack. It was exactly such transference that I saw being played out in the interactions between my father and his admirers.

But it is not only parental or authority figures who become the object of our need for heroes. In our fame-obsessed culture, *anyone* who has achieved celebrity becomes the object of transference, regardless of the reason for his or her renown. We have come to equate fame with the possession of special powers that were once ascribed to gods and mythical heroes. To become widely known is to have achieved a special status in the universe.

Not only do we grant the celebrity a special importance, but we also seek to gain in cosmic stature through our contact with him. In the words of Alan Harrington, "I am making a deeper impression on the cosmos because I know [or have even encountered] this famous person. When the ark sails, I will be on it." The more powerful our idols seem, the more of their magic rubs off on us.

This accounts for the mysterious excitement my father generated in almost any room full of people, all of whom waited eagerly to interact with him. And though I have found it puzzling that others deified my father, I have found myself just as vulnerable to the magic of fame when confronted with celebrities other than he. When I was introduced to Jackie Kennedy a year or two after JFK's death, I was barely able to speak—an almost out-of-body experience. And not so many years ago, when I thought I was about to meet James Taylor, my mouth went dry, and my heart thumped uncontrollably while my brain was telling me, "This is ridiculous! You *know* this is ridiculous!" I knew only too well, but I was overwhelmed by psychological forces beyond my control.

So I am fully appreciative of the power of celebrity and have no illusions that I am more immune to its magic than anyone else. I doubt that we, as a species, can live without the element of excitement and fascination—and, most of all, the illusion of safety—that the idolization of our fellow human beings affords. And so we must acknowledge the full complexity of this issue.

When we project power and authority onto others, we create a reality in which we feel safe enough not only to survive the terrors of the human condition but also to survive them *creatively:* to learn, to grow, to expand our relationship to the world, and to discover ourselves. This is true from earliest childhood, when our exaggerated sense of our parents' capabilities provides the illusion of safety we need to begin to develop as human beings. And throughout our lives, our idealization of teachers, mentors, doctors, religious, and political leaders plays an essential part in our pursuit of both security *and* self-fulfillment. When a person merges with a self-transcending other, Becker writes, "he is, in some real sense, trying to live in some larger expansiveness of meaning. We miss the complexity of heroism if we fail to understand this point.... "

When the object of transference idealization is a man of my father's extraordinary humanitarian vision, wisdom, and compassion, the benefit to others of idolizing and identifying with him is only too obvious. Many have benefited immeasurably from embracing him as a mentor and guide in their pursuit of self-realization. Nevertheless, there is a hidden cost to such idealization: for all the life-enhancing potential of putting our heroes on pedestals, from which their power over us is enhanced, there is also the danger of *self-restriction* in our longing to keep them there. I was constantly struck by the way very successful and competent adults diminished their *own* sense of importance in the presence of my father in the service of magnifying *his*. When we grant another person the status of hero, we instinctively minimize our own virtues and strengths to protect his claim to superiority.

Fromm writes of the fundamental cost of seeking an illusion of safety in this way. He argues that it is ultimately the realization of our own uniqueness and personal integrity that can provide us with the most genuine sense of security in an insecure world. Suspending our belief in ourselves to maintain an illusion of safety in the "other" actually heightens our anxiety and our feelings of helplessness.

When we give ourselves over to the idolization of celebrities, the cost to our sense of ourselves is evident in the way we devalue our own, less celebrated lives. It is easy to fall prey to the myth that fame and *only* fame can provide all the things we want most and bring us ultimate happiness. This devaluation of the nonheroic life permeates our culture and has been brought home to me by the assumptions people continually make about my father and the enchanted life his fame must have brought not only to him but also to all of us close to him. The tragedy is that such illusions can distract us from the genuine gratifications of everyday living, of discovering more about ourselves, of intimate relationships, and of meaningful work.

As much as the glorification of our heroes can provide the conditions essential for our own personal growth, it can also ultimately inhibit the lifelong struggle to separate and individuate—to become increasingly aware of our own unique attributes and strengths and to acknowledge our own power. Obsessing about other (more renowned) people's lives can distract us from celebrating our own lives.

What is often outside of our conscious awareness is the only-too-natural resentment we feel at the *self-sacrifice* inherent in our idealization of others. Just as children feel anger at having to submit to the authority of their caretakers, it is inevitable that we feel resentment at the trade-off we have made when we idealize another human being: diminishing our belief in ourselves to protect our dependent status in relation to him or her. How could we not envy that person's perceived superiority?

An undercurrent of envy is always evident in the way the public relates to celebrities. When we bask in the security of idealized public images, looking to the celebrated for cosmic reassurance and for clues as to how we should try to be, resentment of our lesser status lurks just below the surface. Whenever one of our idols is revealed in a degrading light—exposed for his or her human frailties—what is unleashed is both anger that our idealization has been betrayed and also the resentment that we have almost inevitably felt at our culturally assigned and self-perceived inferiority to that person. Fully aware of this powerful undercurrent and the resulting public thirst for blood, the media attack the fallen like sharks, and we revel in the carnage. For a moment, we feel ourselves to be quite superior after all—our relative unimportance in the universe transformed into relative *importance,* and our lives ennobled by the disgrace of the fallen one.

In truth, however, the only real and enduring liberation from dependency on idealized images lies in our becoming more *aware* of our dependency and of the ways in which it affects our growth. "What makes transference heroics demeaning," Becker writes, "is that the process is unconscious and reflexive, not fully in one's control." While there is little possibility that such primordial processes can ever be *fully* in our control, it is possible to bring the pervasive influence of transference *more* under our control, freeing us to become increasingly self-aware and to accept more responsibility for our own well-being. One medium for exploring this deep personal terrain (and the one I have chosen) is, of course, psychoanalysis, where transferential processes are made the constant focus of attention, with the object of bringing transference distortion as fully as possible to light. After many years of participating in the analytic process (as a patient and as an analyst), I am convinced that, as profoundly important as this self-exploration is for personal growth, nothing can free us *entirely* from our need for transference figures. Our reliance on them is too deeply embedded in our very nature as human beings. Nevertheless, we *can* continue to examine our idealizations and the ways in which they may be inhibiting rather than encouraging our growth. And our strongest ally in this endeavor is our (often covert) anger at the ways in which our exaggerated belief in the power and importance of others deprives us of ourselves.

Even as I write these words, I am deeply engaged in the very struggle I describe. Never have I been more aware of my longing for security in the idealization of others than in the writing of this book. Dreams of isolation, abandonment, and intense loneliness remind me often that, in this writing, I am not only challenging my childhood ties with the most powerful figures in my life—my (now internalized) parents—but I am also offering myself up to be judged on a much wider scale (and potentially more harshly) than ever before. Periods of clarity in the writing have been followed by periods of depression and confusion. And during these difficult times, I have relied heavily on my own mentors to bolster my courage—even as I write about the importance, for all of us, of examining our dependency on such authority figures. Clearly, this is not a story about how I have freed myself from the problem I describe. It is an account of how I have chosen to work at it.

Notes

Chapter 1: Fame and the Fairy Tale

Page

7 **"a universe in miniature":** Max Luthi, *Once Upon a Time: On the Nature of Fairy Tales* (Bloomington: Indiana University Press, 1976), p. 25.
7 **"gold and jewels":** Luthi, *Once Upon a Time*, p. 8.
4 **"beautiful, wise and fortunate":** *The Complete Grimm's Fairy Tales* (New York: Pantheon Books, 1944), p. 8.
5 **"we [too] can become kings and queens":** Jack Zipes, *When Dreams Came True: Classical Fairy Tales and Their Tradition* (New York: Routledge, 1999), p. 7.
5 **"presenting ... polarities of character":** Bruno Bettelheim, *The Uses of Enchantment: The Meaning and Importance of Fairy Tales* (New York: Vintage Books, 1989), p. 9.

Chapter 2: The Orinda Years

Page

12 **This unpredictability:** Conversation with Linn Baldwin Underhill, December 21, 2000.
12 **"terrified to be alone with Erik":** Conversation with Ann Baldwin Williams, December 3, 2000.
16 **"I didn't have a chance":** Conversation with Martha Procter, November 10, 2000.
17 **One childhood friend remembers:** Conversation with Ann Baldwin Williams, December 3, 2000.
18 **told us Neil died to protect us:** Lawrence J. Friedman, *Identity's Architect: A Biography of Erik H. Erikson* (New York: Scribner, 1999), p. 209.
18 **considered divorce:** Friedman, *Identity's Architect*, p. 211.
19 **Some years later:** Conversation with Linn Baldwin Underhill, March 31, 2001.
20 **Our friends the Baldwins:** Conversations with Linn Baldwin Underhill, December 21, 2000, and Ann Baldwin Williams, December 3, 2000.
20 **"terribly unhappy":** Conversation with Ann Baldwin Williams, December 3, 2000.
21 **So one day [she] prevailed:** One of a series of reminiscences written by my mother when she was in her eighties.
22 **how much my parents did for her:** Conversation with Margaret Gompertz Huntington, October 4, 1997.

Chapter 3: My Parents' Childhoods

Page

29 "He would have been nothing": Friedman, p. 86, and conversation with Ruth Hirsch, August 16, 2001.
30 "All through my earlier childhood": Erik H. Erikson, *Life History and the Historical Moment* (New York: W. W. Norton, 1975), p. 27.
30 "Do you know who your father is?": Betty J. Lifton, *Journey of the Adopted Self: A Quest for Wholeness* (New York: Basic Books, 1994), p. 205.
31 "Adoption was the great theme": Lifton, *Journey of the Adopted Self,* p. 66.
31 "If my father hadn't cared": Lifton, *Journey of the Adopted Self,* p. 206.
31 "The unnaturalness of not knowing": Lifton, *Journey of the Adopted Self,* p. 67.
31 "There is the presumption": Lifton, *Journey of the Adopted Self,* p. 71.
31 "If the malignancy": Erikson, *Life History,* p. 31.
31 "anything but the proverbial stepfather": Erikson, *Life History*, p. 27.
32 "Brandes, Kierkegaard, Emerson": Erik H. Erikson, "Autobiographic Notes on the Identity Crisis," *Daedalus* 99, No. 4 (Fall, 1970), p. 745.
32 first male role models: Erikson, "Autobiographic Notes on the Identity Crisis," p. 742.
33 "an adoptive father": Lifton, *Journey of the Adopted Self,* p. 205.
34 "referred to as 'goy'": Erikson, *Life History,* p. 27.
34 "My sense of being 'different'": Erikson, *Life History.*
35 "intensely alienated": Erikson, *Life History*, p. 28.
35 mediocre grades: Friedman, p. 43.
35 "I will not describe": Erikson, *Life History,* p. 26.
36 "It must be more obvious now": Erikson, *Life History*, p. 29.
36 "Oh, well, Margaret": Margaret Brenman-Gibson, "The Legacy of Erik Homburger Erikson," *The Psychoanalytic Review,* 84, No. 3 (June 1997), p. 331.
36 A "habitual stepson": Erikson, "Autobiographic Notes," p. 744.

Chapter 4: They Meet

Page

40 "You big man now": Erik H. Erikson, *Childhood and Society* (New York: W. W. Norton, 1950), p. 147.
44 "never acquired an abiding interest": Friedman, p. 86.
45 "cultivate not-belonging": Erikson, *Life History,* p. 29.
45 saved his life: Friedman, p. 56.
45 Peter suspected: Conversations with Peter Blos on March 7, 1995, and November 14, 1995.
45 "family romance": Friedman, p. 87.
46 Dad needed a male therapist: Friedman.

Chapter 6: Berkeley in the 1960s

Page

62 "depicts over and over": Luthi, p. 140.

Chapter 7: New Beginnings

Page

80 erroneously stereotyped: Friedman, p. 425.
80 "built on systematic repression": Marshall Berman, *New York Times Book Review,* March 30, 1975, pp. 1–2.
81 "not wholly off the mark": Friedman, p. 432.
81 sales of his books plummeted: Friedman, p. 434.

Chapter 8: Becoming a Psychoanalyst

Page

87 "a very bright and able scholar": Robert Coles, *Erik H. Erikson: The Growth of His Work* (Boston: Little, Brown, 1970), pp. 259–60.
89 the "relational" perspective: Sypros D. Orfanos, "Relational Psychoanalysis," *Encyclopedia of Psychotherapy,* Vol. 2 (Elsevier Science [USA], 2002).

Chapter 9: Laurence Olivier

Page

93 My fascination with Laurence Olivier: Barbara Walters interview of Laurence Olivier, ABC, October 10, 1983.
94 Olivier's *Confessions*: *Confessions of an Actor* (New York: Penguin Books, 1984).
94 "You have weakness ... *here*": *Confessions of an Actor*, pp. 37–38.
94 insisted on using nose putty: *Confessions of an Actor*, p. 38.
94 "I have always had that rod of steel": Laurence Olivier, *On Acting* (New York: Simon & Schuster, 1987), p. 192.
95 a "sense of slight disgust": Olivier, *Confessions*, p. 18.
95 "that sidey litde shit": Olivier, *Confessions*, p. 31.
95 "the wish for this treacherous glory": Olivier, *Confessions,* p. 30.
95 "My will was granite": Olivier, *On Acting,* p. 141.
96 "An actor must act": Olivier, *On Acting*, p. 85.

Chapter 10: The Quest for Understanding

Page

97 Eleanor Roosevelt's mother: Eleanor Roosevelt, *The Autobiography of Eleanor Roosevelt* (New York: De Capo Press, 1961), pp. 9–13.
97 Mikhail Baryshnikov's mother: Bruce Glassman, *Mikhail Baryshnikov: Dance Genius* (Woodbridge, CT: Blackbirch Press, 2001), p. 10.
97 Louis Armstrong was abandoned: Laurence Bergreen, *Louis Armstrong: An Extravagant Life* (New York: Broadway Books, 1998), p. 16.
97 Napoleon was sent away: Alan Schom, *Napoleon Bonaparte* (New York: HarperCollins, 1998), p. 1.
97 Virginia Woolf was a victim: Louise DeSalvo, *Virginia Woolf: The Impact of Childhood Sexual Abuse on Her Life and Work* (New York: Ballantine Books, 1990), pp. 1–15.
97 Charles Lindbergh was conscripted: A. Scott Berg, *Lindbergh* (New York: Berkley Books, 1999), pp. 27–53.

98 Maya Angelou retreated into books: Maya Angelou, *I Know Why the Caged Bird Sings* (New York: Bantam Books, 1971), p. 13.

98 bought an old movie camera: Agnes Varda, director, *Jacquot de Nantes,* 1991, a film tribute to her late husband, Jacques Demy.

98 a confirmed "darkroom monkey": Jonathan Spaulding, *Ansel A dams and the American Landscape* (Berkeley: University of California Press, 1998), p. 28.

98 "the people in books were more real": James Baldwin, blurb on the back jacket of Maya Angelou, *I Know Why the Caged Bird Sings* (New York: Bantam Books, 1971).

98 "... when Louis Armstrong wailed": *CBS News Sunday Morning,* "Celebrating Satchmo's Centennial," July 1, 2001.

99 Amelia Earhart's father: Mary S. Lovell, *The Sound of Wings: The Life of Amelia Earhart* (New York: St. Martin's Press, 1989), p. 15.

99 Charlie Chaplin's mother: Charles Chaplin, *My Autobiography* (New York: Plume, 1992), p. 41.

100 the connection between *shame* ... and *grandiosity*: Andrew P. Morrison, *Shame: The Underside of Narcissism* (Hillsdale, NJ: The Analytic Press, 1989); Andrew P. Morrison, "Shame, Ideal Self, and Narcissism," in Morrison, ed., *Essential Papers on Narcissism* (New York: New York University Press, 1986), pp. 348–71; Helen Block Lewis, "Shame and the Narcissistic Personality," in Donald Nathanson, ed., *The Many Faces of Shame* (New York: The Guilford Press, 1987), pp. 93–132; Alice Miller, "Depression and Grandiosity as Related Forms of Narcissistic Disturbances," in Morrison ed., *Essential Papers,* pp. 323–47.

100 W.R.D. Fairbairn was one of the first: W.R.D. Fairbairn, "The Repression and the Return of Bad Objects," in Peter Buckley, ed., *Essential Papers on Object Relations* (New York: New York University Press, 1986), pp. 102–26.

101 Alice Miller's classic book: Alice Miller, *The Drama of the Gifted Child: The Search for the True Self* (New York: Basic Books, 1981).

102 "I could never doubt": Erikson, *Life History*, p. 31.

102 *Yo el Rey*: Norman Mailer, *Portrait of Picasso as a Young Man* (New York: Warner Books, 1996), p. 5.

102 decided for him by his mother: Meryle Secrest, *Frank Lloyd Wright* (New York: Knopf, 1992), p. 58.

103 "Work is life for me": Olivier, *Confessions*, p. 39.

103 "monomaniacal preoccupation": Dean Keith Simonton, *Greatness: Who Makes History and Why* (New York: The Guilford Press, 1994), pp. 140–41.

104 "most happy when I'm on stage": "Faces of Elaine Paige," Bravo Cable Network, November 1996.

Page

104 "it is only in his work": Tennessee Williams, "The Catastrophe of Success," *The Glass Menagerie* (New York: New Directions, 1947), p. 14.

104 "The main thing": Leo Braudy, *The Frenzy of Renown: Fame and Its History* (New York: Oxford University Press, 1986), p. 10.

104 the love of the audience: Otto Fenichel, "On Acting," *The Psychoanalytic Quarterly,* Vol. 15 (1946), p. 148.

105 "Good baby": *CBS News Sunday Morning,* "Jerry Lewis: Always 9," May 20, 2001.

105 "I was an orphan": *CBS News Sunday Morning,* interview with Eartha Kitt, April 30, 2000.

105 "This need for another self": *CBS News Sunday Morning,* "Going Home with John Updike," June 11, 2000.

Chapter 11: Going Public Myself

Page

108 "the public Somebody you are": Williams, p. 16.
110 "What is all the fuss about?": Olivier, *On Acting*, p. 233.
111 "I had grandiose plans": Sarah Boxer, "So, Woody, Do You Feel Like Talking About It?," *NewYork Times,* November 11, 2002, p. E5.
111 he was not "taken seriously": "Leonard Bernstein: Reaching for the Note," WNET American Masters Series, 1998, Susan Lacy, producer.
112 "All I hear these days": Brenman-Gibson, "Legacy of Erik Homburger Erikson," p. 334.
112 he was soon overwhelmed: Olivier, *Confessions*, pp. 306–09.
115 an important biography: Friedman.
116 It was suggested: Sue Erikson Bloland, "Fame: The Power and Cost of a Fantasy," *The Atlantic Monthly*, November 1999, pp. 51–62.

Chapter 12: The Eye of the Beholder

Page

118 "*Homo sapiens*, standard vintage": Ernest Becker, *The Denial of Death* (New York: The Free Press, 1973), pp. 128–33.
114 the "ultimate rescuer defense": Irvin D. Yalom, *Existential Psychotherapy* (New York: Basic Books, 1980), p. 129.
118 escape from "freedom": Erich Fromm, *Escape from Freedom* (New York: Avon Books, 1965), p. 163.
119 "When the ark sails": Alan Harrington, *The Immortalist* (Berkeley: Celestial Arts, 1977), p. 101.
119 When we project power: Becker, p. 157.
119 When a person merges: Becker, p. 152.
121 "What makes transference heroics demeaning": Becker, p. 156.

Index

For Product Safety Concerns and Information please contact our EU
representative GPSR@taylorandfrancis.com
Taylor & Francis Verlag GmbH, Kaufingerstraße 24, 80331 München, Germany

www.ingramcontent.com/pod-product-compliance
Ingram Content Group UK Ltd.
Pitfield, Milton Keynes, MK11 3LW, UK
UKHW021517181026
476628UK00015B/524
9781041084167